Living in the Garden of Eden

Robert Abel

Valentine Publishing House
Denver, Colorado

Valentine Publishing House
P.O. Box 27422
Denver, Colorado 80227

This book is not intended as a substitute for medical advice. The reader should consult a physician or medical practitioner in all matters of health and symptoms that may require diagnosis or medical treatment.

The Scripture quotations contained herein are from the *New Revised Standard Version Bible,* copyright © 1989 by the Division of Christian Education of the National Council of the Churches of Christ in the U.S.A. Used by permission. All rights reserved.

Publisher's Cataloging-in-Publication Data
    Abel, Robert.
    Living in the Garden of Eden / Robert Abel.

    p. : ill. ; cm.

    ISBN–10: 0-9796331-4-1
    ISBN–13: 978-0-9796331-4-0

    1. Christian healing.
    2. Natural food diet.
    3. Environmental health. I. Title.

    R733.A527 2016
    615.5—dc21

Printed in the United States of America.

God made the two great lights—the greater light to rule the day and the lesser light to rule the night—and the stars. God set them in the dome of the sky to give light upon the earth, to rule over the day and over the night, and to separate the light from the darkness. And God saw that it was good.

Genesis 1:16–18

Table of Contents

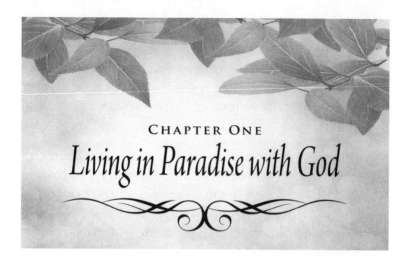

CHAPTER ONE

Living in Paradise with God

In the beginning when God created the heavens and the earth, the earth was a formless void and darkness covered the face of the deep, while a wind from God swept over the face of the waters. Then God said, "Let there be light"; and there was light. And God saw that the light was good; and God separated the light from the darkness. God called the light Day, and the darkness he called Night. And there was evening and there was morning, the first day. ~ Genesis 1:1–5

According to Genesis 1:6–8, God said, *"Let there be a dome in the midst of the waters, and let it separate the waters from the waters." So God made the dome and separated the waters that were under the dome from the waters that were above the dome. And it was so. God called the dome Sky. And there was evening and there was morning, the second day.*

When God finished creating the dome of water above the earth's atmosphere, the sunlight would sparkle through the *waters that were above the dome*[1] during the day almost like the ocean's ripples through a crystal-clear tide on a white sandy beach. The waters above the dome also provided a soft luminescent glow in the evening twilight. At night, ripples of light would reflect through the waters, creating a sense of peace and tranquility.

Because of the dome's ability to increase barometric pressure, it also increased the amount of oxygen that was available to every living organism on the planet. The lush tropical plants in the Garden of Eden would grow to an enormous size. The dome would also create a greenhouse effect, allowing for perfect humidity and temperature throughout paradise. It would be like living on a tropical island with constant 80-degree temperatures, except only better.

The fact that Adam and Eve enjoyed more oxygen in the air has also been established through fossil records. When scientists find pockets of air trapped inside amber (fossilized tree sap) or pockets of air from Antarctica ice-core samples, there's always a greater percentage of oxygen in the air from the past (approximately 35 percent oxygen) compared to what we are currently breathing today (about 20 percent oxygen).

Another benefit of having a dome of water above the stratosphere would be its ability to filter out the sun's harmful ultraviolet rays. In our current environment, overexposure to the sun's ultraviolet rays has the ability to damage the DNA within our skin cells. When the cell's ability to read its own genetic code is hindered, it's possible for that cell to mutate, take on a life of its own and become cancerous.

A cell with defective DNA will no longer interact with the other cells in the human body according to its genetic programming, and when this happens, the rebellious cells can start metabolizing sugars to live longer. When enough cancerous cells grow together, tumors are formed, and when given enough time, they can spread to other parts of the body. A good example of this is melanoma, a deadly form of skin cancer that's caused by prolonged exposure to the sun's ultraviolet rays. When left untreated, melanoma can spread to the brain or lungs and become fatal.

When scientists attempt to recreate similar atmospheric conditions that existed in the Garden of Eden, the results are amazing. In one hyperoxic chamber, scientists increased oxygen levels to 31 percent and were able to spawn dragonflies with bodies 15 percent larger than those that live in our current environment.[2] One group of dragonflies grew normal wingspans of about 3.5 inches, while those that received more oxygen produced four-inch wingspans.

More oxygen in our atmosphere would also allow people to live longer, healthier lives. That's because oxygen is the most important molecule in the human body. Our bodies are comprised of mostly water, and water is comprised of two atoms of hydrogen and one atom of oxygen. Because oxygen weighs more than hydrogen, 65 percent of our body's weight is comprised of oxygen, and 90 percent of our biological energy comes from oxygen.

An increased amount of oxygen in our atmosphere would also explain why many of the men in the Old Testament lived longer lives. For example, according to Genesis 5:5, *all the days that Adam lived were nine hundred thirty years.* According to Genesis 5:22–24, *Enoch walked with God after the birth of Methuselah three hundred years, and had other sons and daughters. Thus all the days of Enoch were three hundred sixty-five years. Enoch walked with God; then he was no more, because God took him.*

An increased amount of oxygen in our atmosphere would also have the ability to prevent disease, because disease-causing viruses, bacteria and pathogens cannot survive in an oxygen-rich environment. A good example of how an oxygen-rich environment can prevent disease comes from the human body's ability to make its own hydrogen peroxide. Hydrogen peroxide is comprised of one water molecule (H_2O) with an extra atom of oxygen (H_2O_2). When hydrogen peroxide comes in contact with a harmful form of bacteria (anaerobic), the extra atom of oxygen is released and the bacteria dies.

A French physician originally discovered oxygen therapy in 1783 after successfully treating a patient that had been suffering from tuberculosis. Since that time, doctors have been treating patients in hyperbaric oxygen chambers. Inside these pressurized chambers, the patients are given 100% oxygen to breathe, and the results have been outstanding. People have been healed of many neurological disorders, including Parkinson's, Alzheimer's and Lou Gehrig's disease.

Perfect Fellowship with God

The Garden of Eden would have been the most lush, beautiful, tropical paradise imaginable. There would have been an abundance of wildlife, large butterflies and purified streams all surrounded by brightly colored flowers and blooming fruit trees. And to make paradise even more incredible, God would personally commune with his beloved children on a regular basis.

According to Genesis 3:8, God used to visit Adam and Eve in *the garden at the time of the evening breeze.* Right before sunset, Adam and Eve would finish their work assignments and spend the evening with God, walking along the stone paths that wove through the lush meadows and flowering hillsides.

Adam and Eve had the opportunity to ask God any questions they wanted and receive an abundance of wisdom, knowledge and understanding. God would personally commune with his beloved children, spending time with them, as they enjoyed each other's company. God would spend countless hours with Adam and Eve, describing all the intricate details of nature and teaching them how to care for his creation.

Then one day everything changed. Eve found herself being seduced by a very seductive and alluring voice. An angelic being that had been previously cast out of heaven many years ago disguised his true identity in the form of a serpent and slithered in the shadows, waiting for an opportunity to strike. When Eve was alone in the garden, the serpent said to her, *"Did God say, 'You shall not eat from any tree in the garden'?"*[3]

Startled by the voice, Eve quickly turned around and said, *"We may eat of the fruit of the trees in the garden; but God said, 'You shall not eat of the fruit of the tree that is in the middle of the garden, nor shall you touch it, or you shall die.'"*[4]

The serpent slowly coiled his camouflaged body into a circle, raised his head off the ground and said, *"You will not die; for God knows that when you eat of it your eyes will be opened, and you will be like God, knowing good and evil."*[5]

Our Fall from Grace

After thinking about what it would be like to obtain supernatural powers, Eve approached the tree in the center of the garden. She noticed that *the tree was good for food, and that it was a delight to the eyes.*[6] Because Eve wanted to become wise, she *took of its fruit and ate; and she also gave some to her husband, who was with her, and he ate.*[7]

Later that evening, when Adam and Eve heard the sound of the Lord walking in the garden during the time of the evening breeze, they *hid themselves from the presence of the Lord God among the trees of the garden. But the Lord God called to the man, and said to him, "Where are you?"*[8]

Adam was hiding in a patch of tall grass near the cherry orchard. He quickly rose to his feet and said, *"I heard the sound of you in the garden, and I was afraid, because I was naked; and I hid myself."*[9]

"Who told you that you were naked? Have you eaten from the tree of which I commanded you not to eat?"[10]

Then Adam said, *"The woman whom you gave to be with me, she gave me fruit from the tree, and I ate."*[11]

Eve was also hiding in the tall grass near her husband, so the Lord said to her, *"What is this that you have done?"*[12]

"The serpent tricked me, and I ate."[13]

After Adam and Eve had fallen from grace, God said, *"See, the man has become like one of us, knowing good and evil; and now, he might reach out his hand and*

take also from the tree of life, and eat, and live forever"
—therefore the Lord God sent him forth from the garden
of Eden, to till the ground from which he was taken.[14]

According to Genesis 3:24, the Lord *drove out the
man; and at the east of the garden of Eden he placed the
cherubim, and a sword flaming and turning to guard the
way to the tree of life.* After Adam and Eve were sent
forth to start a new life, *the Lord God made garments of
skins for the man and for his wife, and clothed them.*[15]

After Adam and Eve had acquired the ability to discern good from evil, the seductive presence of darkness
was allowed to continue his assault against humanity.
The deadly presence knew that if he could tempt God's
children once, he could do it again. His plan was to
speak very subtle and seductive lies to Adam and Eve's
descendants, for the fallen angel knew that if he could
entice Adam and Eve's need for pleasure, he could pervert their entire way of life.

It didn't take long before the entire world fell
prey to his seductive voice. When humanity began to
multiply on the face of the earth, *the Lord saw that the
wickedness of humankind was great in the earth, and that
every inclination of the thoughts of their hearts was only
evil continually. And the Lord was sorry that he had made
humankind on the earth, and it grieved him to his heart.*[16]

Then one day the Lord said to Noah, *"I have de-
termined to make an end of all flesh, for the earth is filled
with violence because of them; now I am going to destroy
them along with the earth. Make yourself an ark of cypress
wood; make rooms in the ark, and cover it inside and out
with pitch."*[17]

"For my part, I am going to bring a flood of waters on the earth, to destroy from under heaven all flesh in which is the breath of life; everything that is on the earth shall die. But I will establish my covenant with you; and you shall come into the ark, you, your sons, your wife, and your sons' wives with you." [18]

After Noah had finished building the ark according to God's instructions, *the fountains of the great deep burst forth, and the windows of the heavens were opened.* [19] *The flood continued forty days on the earth; and the waters increased, and bore up the ark, and it rose high above the earth. The waters swelled so mightily on the earth that all the high mountains under the whole heaven were covered.* [20]

New Atmospheric Conditions

After the dome of water that was suspended in the stratosphere was released, the earth's atmosphere was forever changed. The air became thinner due to decreased barometric pressure. The greenhouse effect, which provided the perfect tropical environment, had transitioned between two opposite extremes—freezing cold at the poles and extremely hot near the equator.

The new changes in the earth's atmosphere also changed humanity's dietary restrictions. In the days before the flood, Adam and Eve enjoyed a strictly vegetarian diet. God's children were given specific instructions to eat only plants, according to Genesis 1:29–30, when God said, *"See, I have given you every plant yielding seed that is upon the face of all the earth, and every tree with seed in its fruit; you shall have them for food. And to every beast of the earth, and to every bird of the air, and to everything that creeps on the earth, everything that has the breath of life, I have given every green plant for food."*

It was God's original design for humanity to eat only plants. The Garden of Eden produced an abundance of every kind of fruit, vegetable, grain and seed imaginable. Because of the increased oxygen, the pre-flood vegetation produced more amino acids (the building blocks of protein) along with an increased amount of phytonutrients (plant-based nutrients), as well as an abundance of vitamins and minerals.

After the flood, when there was less barometric pressure forcing oxygen into every living cell on the planet, the plants could no longer produce the same amount of nutrients, so God allowed humanity to consume a small amount of animal protein. Permission for humanity to consume animal protein was given to Noah and his sons shortly after the floodwaters subsided.

After Noah and his sons built an altar to worship God, the Lord blessed them by saying, *"Be fruitful and multiply, and fill the earth. Every moving thing that lives shall be food for you; and just as I gave you the green plants, I give you everything. Only, you shall not eat flesh with its life, that is, its blood."*[21]

Another change that occurred after the flood was the number of days that humanity was allowed to live. Before the flood, Adam and Eve's descendants could flourish for hundreds of years in an oxygen-rich environment, but after the flood, God limited our life span to 120 years. According to Genesis 6:3, God said, *"My spirit shall not abide in mortals forever, for they are flesh; their days shall be one hundred twenty years."*

Because there is now less oxygen in our atmosphere, we are more susceptible to sickness and disease. According to the National Cancer Institute, "Approximately 39.6 percent of men and women will be diagnosed with cancer at some point during their lifetime."[22] An estimated 1,600,000 new cases of cancer will be diagnosed in the United States this year, and 580,000 people will die from the disease.

According to the World Health Organization, cancer is the leading cause of death worldwide, and the number of new cases is expected to rise by 70 percent over the next two decades.[23] Around one-third of all cancer deaths are due to behavioral and dietary risks, including high body mass index, low fruit and vegetable intake, lack of physical exercise and exposure to toxic chemicals.

The best solution to deal with these problems would be to recreate the same living conditions that existed in the Garden of Eden. By developing a deeper relationship with the Lord, eliminating stress from your life and recreating the same dietary conditions that existed before the flood, you will be able to return back to a more natural state of living with God in paradise.

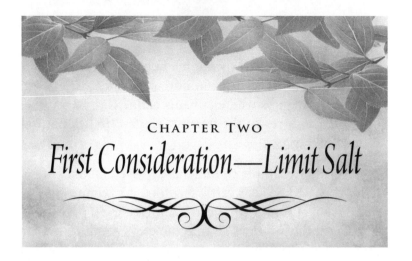

CHAPTER TWO

First Consideration—Limit Salt

The Lord God planted a garden in Eden, in the east; and there he put the man whom he had formed. Out of the ground the Lord God made to grow every tree that is pleasant to the sight and good for food, the tree of life also in the midst of the garden, and the tree of the knowledge of good and evil. ~ Genesis 2:8–9

In the surrounding countryside, deer, bison and cattle roamed freely, feasting on a rich diet of sweet clover, alfalfa and wheatgrass. God's beloved children along with all the animals were able to receive all the nutrients they needed through a natural diet of plants. All of God's creatures lived longer, healthier lives because the pre-flood vegetation contained more phytonutrients, vitamins and minerals than our present-day produce.

Because of the change in our atmosphere, the plants we consume today contain fewer nutrients. As a result, many of God's creatures have either become extinct, live shorter lives or continue to struggle in their efforts to consume a healthy diet. For example, the elephants that lived in the Garden of Eden used to receive all the nutrients they needed through a rich diet of plants, but because of the change in our atmosphere, it's now possible to witness wild elephants eating dirt or traveling long distances to the nearest salt cave to lick natural mineral deposits.

Another example of mineral-deprived animals is dairy cows. In today's cattle feedlots, it's common to find ranchers giving their cattle antibiotics to prevent sickness and hormones so that the cows produce more milk. They also need to place blocks of salt near the animals' water source so they can receive enough sodium. When ranchers fail to offer their cattle blocks of salt, the cows can be observed licking each other or eating strange material such as dirt and wood from the side of the barn.

Sodium-Potassium Ion Exchange

Due to the change in the earth's atmosphere, many people have also experienced problems with their dietary needs. A small amount of sodium is an important nutrient, because it allows the human nervous system to operate properly. Without sodium, it would not be possible for our brains to send electrical impulses to other parts of our bodies. This communication process is called the *sodium-potassium ion exchange*.

When a man's brain sends a command to move his hand, an electronic message travels through a series of nerves. The communication travels from one sodium molecule to a potassium molecule to another sodium molecule, and so forth, until the message reaches its final destination. Without sodium, the human nervous system would not function properly, and without a fully functioning nervous system, both humans and animals would experience extreme difficulties.

Although sodium is a necessary nutrient, it's important to understand the difference between sodium and sodium chloride. Sodium is found in very small quantities in plants, and it's possible for the human body to receive an abundance of sodium by eating plants. Sodium chloride is the scientific name for table salt. Although table salt contains sodium, it does not have the same chemical composition.

Sodium is an Alkali Metal

The human body needs a very small amount of sodium that's found in plants, but it does not need (or want) an overabundance of table salt for several reasons. First of all, sodium in its natural state is a highly volatile alkali metal. When you separate sodium from table salt, you obtain a silvery-white metal that's so soft it can be cut with a butter knife. Sodium in its natural state is also highly volatile and dangerous, because it reacts violently when mixed with water.

It's possible to purchase pure sodium on the Internet for laboratory use. The 25-gram ingots usually come packaged in mineral oil, because when sodium is mixed with water, it produces hydrogen. During this chemical reaction, so much heat is generated that the hydrogen gas spontaneously combusts. When a small piece of pure sodium is dropped in water, it will dance on the surface of the water for a few seconds before bursting into flames. When a large piece of sodium is thrown into a pond, it will create an explosion.

To see just how violently pure sodium reacts with water, it's possible to watch videos on the Internet. All you need to do is conduct a search using the keywords "mixing alkali metals with water." There, you will find six alkali metals from the periodic table that will produce reactions ranging from mild to severe in the following order: lithium, sodium, potassium, rubidium, cesium and francium. For example, when you drop two ounces of cesium in a bathtub of water, it will create an explosion similar to a hand grenade.

Another reason why the human body only wants a very small amount of sodium is because it is poisonous and highly toxic. When a man eats too much table salt, it will make him vomit. When salty water is poured on a plant, it will poison the plant and turn the leaves brown. Table salt is also corrosive and has the ability to rust metal. When you rub salt into a wound, it will burn. Sodium chloride is also the number one cause of heart disease throughout the world, and even though it has the ability to trick a person's brain into thinking that food tastes better, it's responsible for killing millions of people each year.

Hardening of the Arteries

To understand why table salt is so harmful to a person's health, it may be helpful to picture a small flexible plastic tube that represents a man's arteries. It's important for our arteries to remain flexible and free of plaque buildup, just like you would want the garden hose at your home to remain soft, flexible and free from interior blockages.

If we were to pump acid through a plastic tube, the corrosive substance would soften the inner walls and eventually cause a breach. When a man pumps too much salt through his arteries, the corrosive substance has the ability to weaken the elastic fibers.

When a breach occurs inside a man's arteries, his body will quickly repair the damaged area with a patch. When too many patches accumulate over the years, the condition is called *hardening of the arteries.* When this occurs, the man's arteries are no longer soft and flexible but become hardened and brittle, making them more susceptible to future breaches.

Another problem with placing too many patches inside a breached pipe is that plaque can get caught on the repaired surface. Not only will too many patches restrict blood flow, but if one of those patches accumulates a lot of buildup and breaks free, it can travel through the man's arteries. If the debris enters a smaller capillary, it can become lodged, creating a blockage. When plaque blocks the main arteries leading to a person's brain, it can cause a stroke.

When a stroke occurs, the area of the brain with restricted blood flow will stop functioning properly. Stroke victims usually experience dizziness, trouble speaking and weakness as their ability to function becomes impaired. Stroke victims will oftentimes lose balance and fall to the ground unconscious. If a stroke victim does not receive immediate medical attention, the damage can be severe and irreversible.

Cardiovascular Disease

In addition to damaging the cellular integrity of our arteries, eating too much table salt is the number one cause of cardiovascular disease. When a man eats sodium chloride, it causes the cells in his body to swell through the process of osmosis. Although the process of osmosis might not sound so bad, it has a devastating effect on a person's heart, because the heart will have to pump blood through swollen body parts.

When the cells in a man's arms and legs become swollen, they press against his skin, and although his skin can stretch a little, it will constantly press back and transfer the pressure back to his arteries. When a man's heart has to constantly pump blood through swollen body parts, it causes the valves and muscles in his heart to wear out prematurely.

According to the World Health Organization, it is estimated that over 17.5 million people die every year from heart disease.[1] According to a review published in *The New England Journal of Medicine*, consuming too much salt is responsible for more than 1.6 million cardiovascular-related deaths annually.[2]

The human heart has been designed by God to last our entire lifetime. When a man eats too much table salt, it will restrict blood flow in his arteries and place a burden on one of the most important organs in his body. When a person's heart stops beating, they usually die within minutes. Our hearts can never stop to take a rest. They have to continue pumping blood night and day, every second, for as long as we want to live.

The best way to give our hearts a break is to consume a healthy diet of organic fruits and vegetables, enjoy a good amount of cardiovascular exercise and limit our intake of sodium chloride. When a man stops consuming table salt he will feel better, experience fewer headaches and think more clearly. It will even help him experience a more peaceful and productive night's sleep.

One of the main reasons our bodies require rest at night is to remove toxins. When a man stops consuming sodium chloride, his liver and kidneys will have an easier time rebalancing his body's internal chemistry and restoring his proper sodium-potassium ratio. When a man's liver and kidneys have less work to perform at night removing toxins, his internal organs can focus on more important tasks like preventing sickness and disease.

Reprogramming Your Taste for Salt

When Adam and Eve lived in the Garden of Eden, there was no reason for them to consume table salt. God designed plants to contain a very small amount of sodium, and when we consume a healthy diet of plants, we receive all the sodium that our bodies need. The only reason a person would have to consume table salt is taste.

A good example why taste isn't a very logical reason for a person to consume a potentially harmful substance comes from a young boy named Billy who used to drink his own bathwater. Billy even tried promoting the practice to his friends. When the older boys told Billy that it was "nasty" and that he should stop, Billy defended the practice by saying, "But it tastes good." Although Billy may have been attracted to the salty taste in the water, he eventually realized that taste wasn't a very good reason for his actions.

When Billy consumed a small amount of sodium chloride (along with a few other minerals in the water), his taste buds sent an impulse to a part of his brain called the *nucleus accumbens,* a cluster of nerve cells underneath the cerebral cortex. This part of the brain is commonly referred to as the *pleasure center,* because when it's triggered, it releases a neurotransmitter called *dopamine* that allows a person to experience pleasure.

When a man eats food seasoned with a little salt, his brain will tell him that the food is good and that he should eat more. When a man eats a tablespoonful of salt, his tongue will sense a toxic substance and tell him to spit it out. When a man eats a cup of salt, his body will sense the danger, and he may vomit. So even though a little salt has the ability to trick a person's brain into thinking that food tastes better, it has nothing to do with the food at all.

The good news is that in the same way you can trick your brain into thinking that food tastes better with salt, you can also recalibrate your taste buds by eliminating salt from your diet. All you need to do is lower your salt exposure for a few short months, and soon you will be able to enhance your taste for the natural flavors of food. By completely removing sodium chloride from your diet, you will no longer miss the taste, and if you try eating salty foods, you may even experience a distasteful reaction.

Only 1,500 Milligrams Per Day

According to the American Heart Association, a healthy person who is *not* experiencing high blood pressure, diabetes or cardiovascular disease should limit their sodium consumption to 1,500 mg per day.[3] In the event that a healthy person consumes just one tablespoon of soy sauce, it would provide 95 percent of their daily sodium requirements. Many biscuit or pancake mixes contain 800 mg of sodium per serving due to the sodium content of baking soda. An eight-ounce glass of tomato juice contains 700 mg of sodium.

A one-ounce slice of American cheese may look harmless, but it can contain between 330 and 460 mg of sodium. One slice of bread contains 146 mg of sodium. Although 146 mg of sodium might not seem like a large amount, very few people eat just one slice of bread. When a man consumes several slices of bread, along with processed chicken meat, cheese and a dill pickle for lunch, he has already consumed more than three times the amount of sodium than his body needs.

When God created vegetables, he designed them in such a way that they would provide the perfect amount of sodium that our bodies need. For example, one stick of celery contains 32 mg of sodium, while one cup of chopped kale contains 25 mg of sodium. A sweet potato contains 72 mg of sodium, while an orange and banana hardly contain any, less than 1 mg each.

At the opposite extreme, one large dill pickle contains 1,928 mg of sodium along with many other toxic chemicals. The ingredients printed on one popular brand of dill pickles are listed as follows: cucumbers, water, distilled vinegar, salt, calcium chloride, sodium benzoate, polysorbate 80, natural flavors and yellow #5.

The only valuable ingredient in this product is the cucumbers, but in order to receive the nutritional value from a cucumber, you will need to eat it raw. Once you soak a cucumber in a brine solution, it kills all the cucumber's natural phytonutrients, vitamins and enzymes. As soon as the cucumber is cut off the vine, many of the cancer-fighting and anti-inflammatory phytonutrients begin to decompose.

As for the other ingredients listed on the label: *Calcium chloride* has a salty taste and is used by the food processing industry to make products taste saltier without adding any more salt. *Sodium benzoate* is a food preservative that forms a cancer-causing compound (benzene) when mixed with ascorbic acid. *Polysorbate 80* is used as a food emulsifier to prevent the separation of chemicals as the product sits on the shelf. *Natural flavors* could mean almost anything, including any kind of neurotoxin similar to monosodium glutamate. *Yellow #5* is a food coloring that has caused many people to experience allergic reactions, headaches, blurred vision and a multitude of other side effects.

Replacing Processed Foods

You can return back to a more natural state of living in the Garden of Eden by removing the jar of pickles from your refrigerator and replacing it with a fresh, healthy cucumber. A fresh cucumber contains 6 mg of sodium and many other vitamins and minerals that your body needs, including 18 amino acids, vitamin C, vitamin B1, vitamin K, potassium, phosphorus, molybdenum, magnesium and pantothenic acid.

A fresh cucumber also contains many powerful phytonutrients such as lariciresinol, pinoresinol and secoisolariciresinol, which have been shown to reduce the risk of cardiovascular disease as well as fight several forms of cancer, including breast, uterine, ovarian and prostate cancers. Phytonutrients from fresh cucumbers also contain powerful antioxidant and anti-inflammatory properties. The best part of eating a fresh, raw cucumber the way God intended is that you can rest assured it does not contain any cancer-causing chemicals hidden under the term *natural flavors.*

After you have removed some of the salty foods from your home, you may want to consider replacing the contents of your salt and pepper dispensers with organic ginger root powder and cayenne pepper. It would also be possible to purchase several more dispensers and fill those with organic turmeric and garlic powder. That way when you add flavoring to your food, you will be adding some of nature's most powerful cancer-fighting phytonutrients to your diet.

In the event that you are worried about not receiving enough iodine, it's possible to fill one of your spice dispensers with organic kelp powder. Just a tiny pinch of kelp ($1/_{32}$ of a teaspoon) will provide 700 mcg of iodine, or approximately 460 percent of the recommended dietary allowance set by the National Institutes of Health.[4]

You can return back to a more natural state of living in the Garden of Eden by eliminating sodium chloride from your diet. The healthy choice is God's gift to you. It will prevent the hardening of your arteries, alleviate headaches, prevent the unnecessary swelling of every cell in your body, lower your blood pressure, allow your blood to flow more efficiently, reduce the risk of strokes and heart attacks, rejuvenate your internal organs, keep your arteries flexible and prolong your health and well-being.

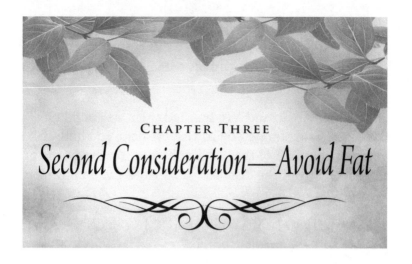

CHAPTER THREE

Second Consideration—Avoid Fat

Because Adam and Eve could no longer live in the garden, they traveled a short distance to the east and began building a home near the stream. Eve was inspired with the idea after watching honeybees construct a hive. She started the work by gathering tree branches, while Adam dug holes in the ground using a flat piece of shale that served as a shovel.

After placing the larger ends of the tree branches in the holes, Adam tied the flexible ends together over the center, forming a dome. To make the structure more secure, Eve wove smaller flexible sticks through the branches and tied the latticework together using vines. While she framed a door opening, along with several windows, Adam prepared a mixture of mud and clay near the stream. Once the wooden structure was complete, Adam covered the branches with a reddish-brown adobe finish.

The home turned out beautifully, and it even enjoyed the protection of several large oak trees growing near the northwest corner. All their new home needed was a cobblestone path leading down toward the stream and several vegetable gardens that Eve was planning for the southern hillside.

After Adam and Eve finished their first building project, God stopped by to visit his beloved children during the time of the evening breeze. As the Lord approached from the distance, Adam and Eve ran to meet him.

"We're so happy you're here," Eve said. "Please come and see our new home."

"It's very nice," God said. "I like how you used palm branches to create the roof."

"Except I couldn't figure out how to attach the top layer," Adam said.

"Rainwater drips down the center pole at night," Eve said.

"Have you tried heating some pine sap to make an adhesive?" God said.

"That's a great idea," Adam said. "I could use fire from the volcano and a large seashell for a container."

"Please be careful near the flowing lava," God said. "There's enough heat near the hot sulfur springs."

"Is there something Adam could heat to make our clothes softer?" Eve said. "The animal skin garments you made for us are a little bit stiff."

"You can soften your clothing by heating animal fat and rubbing the liquid into the leather," God said. "Just be careful when heating fat because it's flammable."

"Can we use fat for any other projects?" Adam asked.

"You may use it to make an oil lamp or for candles to burn at night," God said. "But remember my instructions, you're not allowed to consume any animal fat."

"I have already learned my lesson," Eve said. "I'll never be tempted by food again."

"Very good," God said. "If you walk with me back to the garden, I will share with you why it's harmful to consume animal fat. That way, you can help inform the future generations."

God's Law Concerning Fat

Throughout the generations, it became necessary for God to continue repeating his instructions concerning animal fat. For example, in Leviticus 3:17 the Lord said, *"It shall be a perpetual statute throughout your generations, in all your settlements: you must not eat any fat or any blood."*

In Leviticus 7:23–24 the Lord said, *"You shall eat no fat of ox or sheep or goat. The fat of an animal that died or was torn by wild animals may be put to any use, but you must not eat it."*

After God issued strict laws concerning the consumption of animal fat, a question began to surface regarding how we should interpret those laws. In the same way the serpent asked Eve a very seductive question regarding what God said about eating from the tree in the center of the garden, so too does the question repeat itself again today. "Did God really say that? If so, what do you think it means?" And because animal fat tastes so good and smells so delicious on the barbecue grill, why would God give such a law in the first place?

To answer these questions, it will be helpful to revert back to the Garden of Eden. When the earth's atmosphere contained more oxygen, plants could produce all the healthy omega-3 and omega-6 fatty acids that our bodies needed. For example, one cup of walnuts in our current environment contains 10.6 grams of omega-3 and 44.5 grams of omega-6 fatty acids.

Because the United States Food and Nutrition Board recommends 1.6 grams of omega-3 and 17 grams of omega-6 fatty acids for adult males per day, if a man consumed one cup of walnuts, he would receive 660 percent more omega-3 fatty acids and 260 percent more omega-6 fatty acids than his body needed that day.[1]

The only *essential* fatty acids that the human body needs are monounsaturated and polyunsaturated fat (also referred to as omega-3 and omega-6 fatty acids). These fats are considered *essential* because the human body cannot make them, and they must be consumed in our diet. The human body needs a very small amount of monounsaturated and polyunsaturated fat to construct outer nerve coverings and to build cell membranes.

The difference between monounsaturated and polyunsaturated fats is in their single or double bonding structures. Polyunsaturated fat remains liquid inside the refrigerator, while monounsaturated fat starts to solidify inside the refrigerator.

Saturated Animal Fat

The other type of fat that is considered *nonessential* is saturated fat. The word *saturated* refers to the number of hydrogen atoms surrounding each carbon atom. When the chain of carbon atoms holds as many hydrogen atoms as possible, it becomes *saturated with hydrogen* and remains solid at room temperature. Good examples of foods that contain a high percentage of saturated fat include butter, lard, cream, cheese, pizza, chicken skin, pork, lamb and beef.

One of the main reasons why saturated fat is harmful to our health is that it raises a person's cholesterol levels. There are two types of cholesterol that travel through our arteries. One type called *HDL* (high-density lipoproteins) is considered a good form of cholesterol because it travels around working as a cleaning agent, absorbing the sticky, wax-like animal fat. The other type of cholesterol is called *LDL* (low-density lipoproteins). Although it has a necessary function in making hormones, the human body has the ability to make all the LDL cholesterol that it needs.

When a man consumes saturated animal fat, the amount of bad cholesterol in his blood increases to the point of outnumbering the cleaning agents, and soon the sticky wax-like substance can build up inside his arteries. When plaque accumulates, the interior dimensions of the man's arteries can become constricted and interfere with the flow of blood and oxygen.

When a man experiences a restricted flow of blood in his arteries, it will cause his heart to beat faster and work harder. Because the man's heart can never stop to take a rest, an unnecessary amount of stress over a prolonged period of time will eventually lead to heart disease.

Hydrogenated Vegetable Oil

The other type of fat that is dangerous for human consumption is hydrogenated vegetable oil. The food processing industry also calls hydrogenated vegetable oil *trans fat* or *trans-fatty acid*. Because most vegetables such as corn, palm or safflower are not suitable for cold pressing, they are subjected to chemical processing to extract the oil.

In the case of corn oil, the kernels are milled to separate the germs. Grooved rollers then crush the germs to extract most of the oil. The remaining substance is then treated with hexane to extract the maximum amount of oil. In an attempt to refine the oil and remove any undesirable color and chemical taste, the oil is heated to 180 degrees, mixed with an alkaline solution of sodium hydroxide and sent through a centrifuge. Afterward, the oil is heated in a vacuum at 485 degrees to eliminate any remaining chemical taste.

At this point in the manufacturing process, you have the common vegetable oil that is sold in most grocery stores. In an attempt to give processed foods an even longer shelf life, food manufacturers take the liquid vegetable oil and turn it into a solid using a process called *hydrogenation*.

During the hydrogenation process, vegetable oil is heated in the presence of hydrogen and a heavy metal catalyst, such as nickel or platinum, for the purpose of adding extra hydrogen atoms to the carbon chain. This process can take several hours, but after the molecular structure of the oil has been altered, it will have a higher melting point, and instead of being liquid at room temperature, it becomes semisolid or solid.

The hydrogenation process for vegetable oil is similar to the manufacturing process of plastic, because many types of plastics are created from crude oil. During the plastic manufacturing process, carbon atoms from crude oil are bonded together with hydrogen atoms from water to create long polymer chains. In the same way that hydrogenation can turn crude oil into an indestructible substance that takes hundreds of years to decompose, adding hydrogen atoms to vegetable oil will create an indigestible substance that the human body cannot process.

When a man consumes hydrogenated oils, the chemically modified carbon chains can remain inside his liver for months. Consuming hydrogenated oils will also cause a tremendous burden on a person's internal organs, because the pancreas will keep producing enzymes in an attempt to break down the saturated carbon chains. When the foreign, plastic-like substance circulates throughout a person's arteries, it can trigger false immune responses and place an unnecessary amount of stress on the immune system.

Not only will hydrogenated oil place an enormous amount of stress on a person's internal organs, but the human body needs to construct thousands of new cells per day. The outer walls of a man's cells should be constructed from healthy omega-3 and omega-6 fatty acids so that they function properly. In the event that a man's body doesn't have enough healthy fatty acids to construct all of his cells, his body will use whatever material is available, including modified carbon chains of hydrogenated oils.

When hydrogenated oils are used to construct cell membranes, they can allow pathogens, microbes and other viruses to pass through the cell walls and, at the same time, prevent valuable nutrients from entering. Cell walls that have been constructed from hydrogenated oils can also prevent toxic waste material from exiting. When toxic waste material becomes trapped inside our cells, it can cause the cells to mutate, which may lead to cancer, tumors or other serious health issues.

Fat Cells Store Toxins

Another reason why God doesn't want his beloved children consuming saturated animal fat is because fat cells are designed to store fat-soluble toxins. When a man consumes water-soluble toxins, they are easily flushed from his body via his blood and kidneys, but fat-soluble toxins are more challenging for the body to eliminate. Fat-soluble toxins such as heavy metals, pesticides, preservatives, food additives, pollutants, plastics and other environmental contaminants must become water-soluble for the body to eliminate them.

The fat-soluble detoxification process occurs mostly in the liver, but when the liver becomes overwhelmed with the task of breaking down hydrogenated oils and performing hundreds of other chemical conversions during the day, the fat-soluble toxins usually wait in line for processing. When a person's liver becomes congested with thick bile and an endless supply of toxins, the liver will push those fat-soluble toxins back into the bloodstream. Once toxins enter the bloodstream, the body will either send them back to the liver for processing or store them inside of fat cells.

Animal Fat Contains Toxins

In the same way that humans store toxins in their fat cells, so do animals. In the Garden of Eden, cows could graze freely on the vast meadows of sweet clover, alfalfa and wheatgrass. But in today's cattle feedlots, cows are fed industrial waste. For example, if you live near timber production with sawmills in the area, there's a good chance your local beef supply has been consuming sawdust.

The introduction of sawdust into a cow's diet began the day a farmer noticed his nutrient-deprived cows eating scrap from a nearby paper mill. After making this discovery, he was inspired with the idea of converting sawdust into commercial cattle feed. The only problem was that sawdust is made of cellulose and is bound together with lignin, which makes it hard to digest. To solve this problem, manufacturers began treating sawdust with nitric acid, and today sawdust is commonly used for cattle feed.

Another type of industrial waste that's used for cattle feed is the remains of crab, shrimp and crawfish. Although the internal organs, scales and fins of seafood contain heavy metals, they also provide cattle with a non-vegetarian source of protein. Other industrial waste products that are used to produce cattle feed include chicken poop, which comes with feathers, antibiotics and heavy metals.

Another industrial waste product that cows eat

is chocolate salvage and candy manufacturing waste. Broken pieces of candy and chocolate bars that still contain the plastic wrappers are ground up and fed to cattle in an attempt to fatten them up a few months before they are sold at auction. Other waste products include orange peels, cottonseed and industrial waste from beverage brewers.

In addition to feeding their cattle industrial waste, many ranchers inject their livestock with growth hormones and antibiotics. For example, rBGH is a man-made hormone used to increase a cow's milk production. Although it has been banned in Canada and the European Union, rBGH continues to be used by American dairy farmers since it was approved by the United States Food and Drug Administration in 1994.[2] When cows consume antibiotics, pesticides, heavy metals, pollutants, plastics and other environmental contaminants, the fat-soluble toxins can become trapped in their fat cells, and when we consume animal fat, we are consuming those same toxins.

Saturated Fat Causes Inflammation

A good example of how animal fat causes inflammation and swelling comes from a man named Anthony, who was diagnosed with gout, a painful form of arthritis. Although Anthony was an athletic man in his late forties who maintained a healthy diet, he ate an entire bag of pretzels one day and became dehydrated.

Several days later, he felt a painful sensation in his foot during the night. Because he couldn't sleep, he got out of bed and wrapped his foot in a heating pad. The next morning, the painful sensation was even more excruciating. It felt as if he had a broken bone, so Anthony went to visit his doctor who took an X-ray. Because the X-ray turned out negative, the doctor prescribed a painkiller called *indomethacin*.

After taking the medication for several days, Anthony's situation didn't seem to be improving, so he started searching the Internet for information about gout. According to Anthony's research, "Gout is a type of arthritis. It occurs when uric acid builds up in a person's blood and causes inflammation in the joints. A diet rich in purines from certain foods can raise uric acid levels in the body, which sometimes leads to gout."

After studying this information, Anthony concluded that if eating foods rich in purines caused a buildup of uric acid to settle in his joint, then all he needed to do was stop eating foods rich in purines; and after drinking a lot of water for several days, he should be able to flush the excess uric acid out of his body and everything would be okay.

In an attempt to find out which foods were high in purines, Anthony discovered that 100 grams of sardines contained 480 mg of purines, a beef fillet contained 110 mg, and a chicken breast contained 175 mg of purines. At the low end of the scale, 100 grams of tomatoes contained 11 mg of purines, oranges contained 19 mg, almonds had 37mg and pineapple contained 19 mg.

Because all the meat products were high in purines, Anthony decided that he would stop eating meat until his foot healed. As an alternative to eating meat, Anthony visited his local health food store and purchased several pounds of nuts. He bought a bag of salted almonds because they were high in protein. He also purchased salted sunflower seeds because they were on sale, sweetened banana chips and many other snacks that were all high in salt and fat.

After a week had passed, Anthony's foot still wasn't showing any signs of improvement. The doctor had only given him seven days worth of pain medication, which helped a little, but the drugs never addressed the root cause of the problem. To make matters worse, Anthony was scheduled to depart for an international business trip a few days later. To prepare for the trip, Anthony drank a lot of water and continued eating a diet low in purines, but high in salt and fat.

After spending 10 long and painful days abroad, Anthony returned back to America unable to walk. He needed to ask for assistance in the airport and even rode a medical golf cart to get through customs and immigration. The very next day, Anthony set up an appointment to visit a different doctor. After listening very carefully to everything that Anthony had been through, the doctor said, "I'm a 100 percent convinced that you have gout."

"Then why is it only affecting my left foot?" Anthony asked.

"It happens that way with some people," the doctor said. "The good news is there are three medications that modern medicine can offer you."

The first drug that the doctor suggested was the same painkiller that the first doctor had prescribed. Indomethacin works like Tylenol, except with prolonged use, the drug will destroy a person's liver.

The second drug the doctor prescribed was called *Colcrys,* commonly used for gout and also used to treat Mediterranean fever. The doctor didn't know exactly how this medication worked, but he gave some to Anthony anyway, hoping that it would help.

The third drug had the ability to prevent Anthony's body from producing uric acid, but the doctor didn't recommend taking it, because Anthony's body would eventually grow accustomed to the drug and start producing even more uric acid. At that point, a higher dose of the drug would be needed, and eventually, it would lead to a constant battle between Anthony's body and the ever-increasing need for more drugs.

Because Anthony was in a lot of pain, he accepted the doctor's drugs. Although the drugs alleviated some of the pain, they never addressed the root cause of the problem. Because Anthony was desperate to find a cure, he started making phone calls and found a medical lab near his house that performed walk-in blood tests for a very reasonable price.

The first test Anthony ordered was a complete blood count. The second test was to determine the amount of uric acid in his blood. Because Anthony couldn't read the results himself, he called a doctor at the medical lab where the tests were performed and asked for help. The doctor responded by saying, "Have you tried eliminating salt from your diet?"

"What does salt have to do with anything?" Anthony said. "I have never had a problem with salt before."

"Salt makes my feet swell," the doctor said. "It

won't cost you anything to give it a try. In fact, when you stop eating salt for a few months, you won't even miss the taste."

After getting off the phone with the doctor, Anthony began searching the Internet for "salt makes my feet swell." To his surprise, he found a condition called *edema*. According to his sources, "Edema is caused by excessive fluids being trapped inside the body's tissue that causes swelling in the feet, ankles and legs." After making this discovery, Anthony began searching for other causes of inflammation, and to his surprise, he discovered that fat was the number-one leading cause of inflammation.

As Anthony pondered this information, he began to realize what had happened. When he consumed an entire bag of pretzels, he also consumed over 5,800 mg of salt. Because Anthony's body naturally produced uric acid, it could not flush out the normal amounts of uric acid along with all the salt, because his body had become dehydrated. When the excessive amounts of uric acid settled in the joint, it turned into very sharp, razorblade-like crystals.

Once the razorblade-like crystals had formed, his foot needed several months of rest, but instead of allowing his foot to heal, Anthony continued to walk on the swollen joint, causing even more damage. When Anthony stopped eating meat in an attempt to avoid purines, he began consuming even more salt and fat, which caused even more swelling. It was a vicious cycle. The more salt and fat that Anthony consumed to avoid purines, the more it made his foot swell, and the more his foot swelled, the more pain he experienced.

Because Anthony's blood tests showed that his body was producing normal amounts of uric acid, he didn't need to worry about any more crystals forming. The only problem that Anthony was facing now was inflammation and a heavily damaged joint. To obtain the healing that he needed, Anthony stopped taking the doctor's drugs and completely removed salt and fat from his diet.

Anthony was inspired with the idea after reading a warning label on the prescription that said, "Avoid eating grapefruit or drinking grapefruit juice while taking Colcrys." This gave Anthony the idea that he should stop taking Colcrys and start eating a lot more grapefruit. One reason was that grapefruit naturally contains two antioxidants called *polyphenols* and *nootkatone* that break down stored fat and increase the body's fat-burning activities.

As soon as Anthony stopped consuming salt and fat, he noticed a considerable difference. When he went to sleep at night, his joint was still red, swollen and painful. But when he arose the following morning, the swelling had decreased and his joint was less painful. This slight improvement was all the encouragement that Anthony needed to establish the fact that his so-called gout attack was not being caused by an overabundance of uric acid in his blood, but rather, the pain was being caused by inflammation throughout his body.

Anthony's healing process took about a year to complete. As soon as Anthony completely removed salt and fat from his diet, he noticed a considerable reduction in the amount of pain that he was experiencing. He also noticed a considerable difference in his arms, legs and face. Instead of looking bloated all the time, he started to see the definition of his muscles and a thinner contour in his face. As soon as Anthony addressed the root cause of the problem, he made a complete recovery.

Removing Fat from Your Diet

In an attempt to return back to a more natural state of living in the Garden of Eden, you may want to consider removing all nonessential forms of fat from your diet. To begin this process, it will be helpful to remove all commercially processed foods from your home. Any type of food that contains hydrogenated oil is harmful to your health. According to the United States Food and Drug Administration, there are no safe amounts of hydrogenated oil for human consumption.[3] The worst offenders are margarine, snack crackers, chips and cookies.

When shopping for dairy goods, you may want to consider purchasing organic, fat-free products. Fat-free milk has the same amount of calcium and protein as whole milk, the only difference is the fat. The fat in whole milk may taste better, but it will also add additional calories to your diet, and if you like to eat, you may find that those additional calories are better spent consuming fresh fruits and vegetables.

In the event that you are suffering from arthritis, gout or any other type of inflammation, you may want to stop eating cheese all together. Cheese is full of salt and fat. It's not possible to buy cheese without fat, except for imitation cheese, which will contain other, more harmful ingredients such as corn syrup solids, calcium phosphate, xanthan gum, guar gum, sorbic acid and other toxic chemicals.

When purchasing beef, it's always best to purchase organic, grass-fed products. Cows were designed by God to eat grass. When cattle are fed sawdust, chicken poop, corn silage and candy bars, they will store toxins in their fat cells, and when we eat the saturated fat of animals that have been raised in feedlots, the same harmful toxins and growth hormones will enter our own bodies and cause problems to our health.

Oxidized Oils & Free Radicals

Because oils are created from glycerol and fatty acids, when they are exposed to heat they begin to oxidize, break down and become rancid. The point at which oil turns to smoke is called the *smoke point*, and when this occurs, the glycerol within the oil is converted into acrolein. In addition to creating toxic fumes, heating oil past its smoke point will cause the fatty acids to form free radicals.

The term *free radical* is used to describe an incomplete molecule that wants to steal an electron from another molecule. For example, when you boil water, the H_2O molecules will separate and evaporate in the form of steam. Because these molecules are attracted to each other, when they cool down, they will bond back together again to form liquid.

When you heat oil past its smoke point, it breaks apart the molecular structure and creates incomplete molecules that have a need to steal electrons from other molecules in an attempt to complete their outer shells. Incomplete molecules from heated oils are very unstable and react aggressively with other compounds in an attempt to gain their own stability.

When free radicals from cooking oil enter the human body, they will attach themselves to the closest stable molecule in an attempt to steal an electron. When this occurs, another molecule may become unstable and seek to steal an electron from one of its neighbors, thus starting a chain reaction. Once a chain reaction of electron stealing begins inside a cell, it has the ability to permanently damage that cell.

In an attempt to break the electron-stealing cycle, our bodies will use antioxidants that have the ability to lose one of their own electrons without becoming a free radical themselves. The most abundant fat-soluble antioxidant in the human body is vitamin E and the most abundant water-soluble antioxidant is vitamin C.

Because the fatty acids in cooking oils are sensitive to time decay and heat, it's best to consume them directly from nature. For example, the best way to consume olive oil is to eat fresh olives. The second best way to consume olive oil is to buy a bottle of expeller, cold-pressed oil and keep it refrigerated. The worst possible way to consume olive oil is to allow it to sit in your pantry for several years and then heat it past the smoke point in a frying pan. Even though two-year-old olive oil may look okay, smell delicious and prevent an egg from sticking to the side of a pan, it will be loaded with free radicals.

Organic, Expeller-Pressed Oils

When shopping for cooking oil, it's best to purchase organic, expeller-pressed oils that have a high temperature rating. For example, refined almond oil has a smoke point of 460° F. Another excellent product to use for cooking is organic, salt-free butter (330° F). There's also a refined version of butter called ghee (485° F). Although olive oil makes an excellent salad dressing, it has a very low heat rating and a limited shelf life. Other salad dressings that are *not* suitable for high-temperature cooking include sesame oil and walnut oil.

Cooking oils to avoid would include corn, canola, cottonseed and soybean. Canola oil is produced from a genetically modified and poisonous rapeseed plant. Olestra (or the trade name Olean) is manufactured by bonding vegetable oil and sucrose to form a synthetic compound that the human body cannot digest.[4] Crisco contains fully hydrogenated palm oil, monoglycerides and diglycerides. Lard is a hydrogenated form of pig fat.

Because all types of oil have a limited shelf life and break down at high temperatures to form free radicals, you may also want to avoid eating fried foods. All fried foods are high in fat, and when you purchase them in restaurants (or grocery stores), you never know how long the oil has been sitting in the deep fryer. It's possible that the restaurant staff only changes the oil once a year. Or maybe they never change the oil at all and just keep adding more when the levels run low.

Healthy Nuts & Seeds

One of the best ways to make sure you are getting enough high-quality omega-3 and omega-6 fatty acids in your diet is to start consuming flax seeds. Flax seeds are an amazing gift from God that come loaded with powerful antioxidants. They are about the size of a sesame seed with a very hard shell. The valuable nutrients inside one cup of flax seeds compared to several other nuts and seeds are as follows:

One Cup	Omega-3	Omega-6	Protein
Almonds	0.01 grams	17.2 grams	28.3 grams
Cashews	0.08 grams	11.1 grams	26.2 grams
Flax Seeds	38.3 grams	9.93 grams	30.7 grams
Pumpkin Seeds	0.25 grams	28.5 grams	11.9 grams
Sesame Seeds	0.54 grams	30.7 grams	25.5 grams
Sunflower Seeds	0.10 grams	32.2 grams	29.1 grams
Walnuts	10.6 grams	44.5 grams	17.8 grams

Because omega-3 and omega-6 fatty acids are sensitive to oxygenation, God gave flax seeds a very hard shell. If you cook flax seeds, it will damage the fragile omega-3 and omega-6 benefits, and if you eat the seeds whole, they will pass directly through the digestive system and you will not receive any of their benefits. So the best way to consume flax seeds is by storing them in your refrigerator and grinding them in a coffee grinder right before eating them.

One of the best uses for ground flax seeds is salad dressing. Instead of purchasing commercially processed dressing that's loaded with neurotoxins, flavor enhancers and preservatives, you can grind two tablespoons of flax seed in a coffee grinder and sprinkle the powder over your salad. Other options for a more natural type of salad dressing (that includes protein) would include ground pumpkin seeds, sunflower and chia seeds.

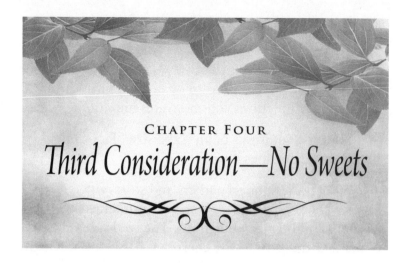

CHAPTER FOUR

Third Consideration—No Sweets

As the evening sun approached the horizon, brilliant rays of yellow and orange transformed the sky into a spectacular spectrum of color as Adam and Eve rested on a large rock with their feet in the stream. They were tired after working all day. The cool water brought about a sense of comfort and joy as they marveled at the sunset while splashing their feet back and forth.

In the distance, they could hear the sound of the Lord approaching, so they ran over to meet him.

"We're so happy you're here," Eve said.

As the Lord approached the couple's home, he said, "I like how you added the shade canopy."

"Thank you," Adam said. "It was Eve's idea."

In the distance, a reddish-brown squirrel was running back and forth along a fallen tree that he was using as a bridge to reach the cherry orchard. As the squirrel traveled the same path, it made Adam wonder. So he asked the Lord, "How does the squirrel know when to harvest cherries?"

"I created squirrels that way," God said. "When the squirrel's brain senses pleasure, it activates his learning and memory functions and motivates him into action."

"But the squirrel's brain is the size of a peanut," Eve said. "How does it work?"

"When the squirrel gathers and stores nuts, it releases a chemical called *dopamine* that interacts with his learning and memory functions. The squirrel is able to remember the path to the cherry orchard, and through hard work, he receives a reward. It's a necessary function of survival that I have given to my creation," God said.

"Wow, that's amazing," Eve said.

"I have also given your brain the same function," God said.

"What do you mean?" Adam asked.

"Come with me," God said, "and I will show you."

As Adam and Eve walked down the cobblestone path leading toward the cherry orchard, God began describing how the pleasure centers of our brains work.

The process is very simple: When a man eats something sweet, his tongue sends a signal to his brain and the brain's pleasure center releases dopamine. This powerful neurotransmitter has the ability to interact with another chemical called *glutamate* to stimulate the man's learning and memory abilities. Because the man can experience the same amount of pleasure eating almonds as he does cherries, there was nothing in God's creation that would cause him to develop a food addiction.

Food addictions occur when we pervert God's creation. God designed fruit to be an excellent source of energy. It's possible for a man to eat three bananas at once, and if he takes one too many bites, his body will tell him "that's enough." After taking the last bite, the man will not think about (or lust after) bananas the rest of the day. That's because God designed bananas with the perfect amount of fiber, glucose, fructose, sucrose, enzymes, vitamins and minerals. Although bananas are sweet, they do not create food addictions.

Food addictions occur when we pervert God's creation. A good example of this comes from ice cream. For example, one pint of Ben & Jerry's New York Super Fudge Chunk contains 220 mg of sodium and 80 grams of saturated fat, which is approximately 125 percent of our recommended dietary allowance.[1] It's also loaded with 1,200 calories and 100 grams of sugar.

When a man buys a pint of his favorite ice cream and takes one bite, his tongue will send a signal to his brain and the brain's pleasure center will release dopamine. As soon as dopamine is released, the man will experience pleasure. In the event that the man eats half the container of ice cream and places the rest in the freezer, his learning and memory center will take note and continually remind him throughout the day that there's still half a container of ice cream available.

When this occurs, the man may find himself thinking about the remaining ice cream all day. His learning and memory center will not stop sending messages to the brain's action center until he goes to the freezer, removes the container and consumes the remaining contents. Once the learning and memory center realizes there's no more ice cream in the freezer, it will stop sending persistent and pestering messages.

Because of the way our brains have been created, it's possible to develop a food addiction to any kind of sweet, salty or fatty food in the same way that it's possible to develop an addiction to marijuana, alcohol or pain pills. That's because our brains only have one pleasure center. The only difference between food addictions and drug addictions is the amount of dopamine that's released. Food addictions trigger our pleasure centers through the natural process of eating, while drugs create a shortcut to the brain's reward center by flooding the nucleus accumbens with dopamine.

Because all man-made sweets will trigger the pleasure center in your brains and release dopamine, the only way to stop tormenting yourself is to completely stop eating them. When you completely remove all man-made sweets from your home and environment, your brain's learning and memory center will take note and stop sending persistent and pestering messages.

Restoring Our Natural Settings

Another way to examine how our brains work would be to picture an internal sweetness thermostat inside your body. When a man eats a healthy diet of fruits, vegetables, grains and seeds (as God intended), then all God's gifts will taste delicious. A man can peel and eat a grapefruit (just like an orange) and it will taste heavenly. His tongue will be able to sense the natural sugars in the grapefruit because his body's internal sweetness thermostat has been set to a very low level.

When a man adds sugar to his grapefruit, his tongue will send a signal to his brain, dopamine will be released, and instantly the grapefruit will taste tart and bitter. That's because the added sugar is comprised of 97 percent sucrose, and it has the ability to raise the man's sweetness thermostat to a higher level. Once the man's sweetness thermostat has been increased to a higher level, he will start craving sweeter foods.

A good example of how this analogy works comes from a man named Bill who had completely eliminated all man-made sweets from his diet. Although Bill was feeling great and had lost a lot of weight, he continued holding on to a large container of honey. Bill didn't consider honey to be a man-made sweetener because it came directly from nature. Bill was only using the honey once a week on the day he worked out at the gym.

When Wednesday morning rolled around, Bill would start the day by eating some fresh fruit and making a large bowl of oatmeal. Next, he would eat half the bowl of oatmeal without any sweetener—then as a special treat to give himself more energy at the gym—he would grab the bottle of honey and drizzle it all over. The honey tasted so delicious that it instantly triggered the pleasure center in his brain. After Bill's brain was flooded with dopamine, he would head off to the gym and work out for two hours.

Although Bill was able to burn off the extra calories that the honey added, he could feel a constant craving for more sweets the rest of the day. When he ate a banana after his workout, it didn't seem as sweet as usual. He also felt more irritable and jittery the rest of the day, as if he had less patience. After noticing how just a little bit of honey affected his cravings and attitude, Bill eventually removed the bottle of honey from his home.

After completely eliminating all sweets from his diet, Bill felt much better. His body didn't need any extra calories, and the brief moment of pleasure that he experienced after eating honey wasn't worth several days of cravings and torment afterward.

Diabetes is a Deadly Disease

Another reason to remove sweets from your diet is to prevent diabetes. In order to understand how diabetes is able to destroy so many people's lives, it will be helpful to start with how the human digestive system works. When a man eats fresh fruits, vegetables, grains and seeds, his digestive system will break down the carbohydrates into glucose. In order for a man's cells to utilize glucose as energy, his pancreas needs to make insulin.

Insulin works like a key that unlocks the door of the cells so that they can receive glucose for energy. In the event that a man's pancreas cannot make enough insulin, or if his pancreas makes poor-quality insulin, his cells will not receive the energy they need to survive. When a man's cells can't receive energy, they begin to die and cause very serious health issues. For example, when the very sensitive cells in a man's eyes become starved for glucose, his vision may become blurry.

When a man consumes a healthy diet of fresh fruits, vegetables, grains and seeds, a steady flow of glucose will enter his bloodstream. Because the man's pancreas was designed by God to last his entire lifetime, it can keep up with the workload and produce the proper amount of high-quality insulin. When the man eats sweets, a flood of glucose will enter his bloodstream and cause his pancreas to work overtime. When the man's pancreas works overtime in an attempt to offset his spiking blood sugar levels, it can grow tired with old age, wear out and begin to malfunction.

When a man's pancreas malfunctions and he cannot produce enough high-quality insulin, he is usually diagnosed with type-two diabetes. When a man's pancreas cannot produce any effective insulin, he is usually diagnosed with type-one diabetes. Both forms of diabetes are extremely serious, and even though they are treatable with a constant supply of insulin, it's always best to prevent the disease from occurring in the first place by eliminating sweets from your diet.

One of the first warning signs for diabetes is excessive thirst and frequent urination. When there's too much unused glucose in a man's bloodstream, his kidneys will try to remove it by extracting water from his blood, which will cause excessive thirst and lead to frequent urination. Another warning sign includes blurry vision. When the very delicate and sensitive cells in a man's eyes can't receive the energy they need, it will affect his ability to focus and can lead to prolonged vision problems and even blindness.

Another warning sign includes extreme fatigue. Even though a man may be eating a lot of high-energy, sugary snacks, if his cells are not receiving the energy they need because his pancreas can no longer produce insulin, he may feel constantly tired. Other symptoms include tingling or numbness in the outer extremities. When a man's body does not have enough insulin to keep his cells alive, it will use the available resources to keep his internal organs functioning, while the outer extremities are usually the first to suffer.

God's Gift of Sweetness

Because the human body has the ability to make all the glucose it needs from a healthy diet of fruits, vegetables, grains and seeds, there's no reason to eat man-made sweets. All forms of man-made sweeteners are destructive to a person's health. Fruit on the other hand is God's gift of sweetness to humanity. When God designed fruit, he carefully formulated the nutrients so that they would never harm his beloved children's bodies or cause food addictions.

One of God's best design elements in fruit is high fiber content. Because fruit offers a lot of healthy fiber, it also has the ability to make a person feel full. The high amount of fiber in fruit also determines how quickly the digestive system will break down the sugars. Because fruit is rich in natural fibers, it helps slow down the absorption of glucose in the bloodstream.

Another brilliant design element that God used when creating fruit is the different variation of sugars. Fruit contains three different types (glucose, fructose and sucrose) that are metabolized in different ways. For example, when a man eats 100 mg of sweet cherries, 8.1 mg of glucose will enter his bloodstream where it can be used by every cell in his body.

Because fructose can *only* be processed by the liver, when a man eats 100 mg of sweet cherries, 6.2 mg of fructose will enter his liver and be converted into a fatty acid. The good news is that the fatty acid will be available for his body to use several hours after eating the cherries. The bad news is that if the man's body doesn't need any additional energy, the fatty acid will eventually be converted into saturated fat.

Because sucrose is a combination of both glucose and fructose, the human body will use an enzyme called *beta-fructosidase* to separate sucrose into its individual units of glucose and fructose. After the separation occurs, the glucose can be used by every cell in the body, while the fructose will be sent to the liver to undergo the fatty acid conversion process.

Although *natural* sweeteners may seem like a healthy alternative to *man-made* sweeteners, they have the ability to cause the same amount of cravings and damage to a person's pancreas because of their high glucose, fructose and sucrose levels.

The following chart shows the sugar content per 100 mg of sweetener:

Sweetener	Glucose	Fructose	Sucrose
White Sugar	0 mg	0 mg	97 mg
Brown Sugar	3.2 mg	2 mg	84.1 mg
Maple Syrup	6.2 mg	1.8 mg	72 mg
Molasses	11.2 mg	12.9 mg	34.7 mg
Honey	33.8 mg	42.4 mg	1.5 mg
Guava Nectar	12.5 mg	74.8 mg	0 mg
Fructose Corn Syrup	7.2 mg	78 mg	0 mg

In comparison, the following chart shows the sugar content per 100 mg of fruit:

Fruit	Glucose	Fructose	Sucrose
Apple	2.3 mg	7.6 mg	3.3 mg
Banana	4.2 mg	2.7 mg	6.5 mg
Grapefruit	1.3 mg	1.2 mg	3.4 mg
Mango	0.7 mg	2.9 mg	9.9 mg
Papaya	1.4 mg	2.7 mg	1.8 mg
Pineapple	2.9 mg	2.1 mg	3.1 mg
Sweet Cherries	8.1 mg	6.2 mg	0.2 mg

Artificial Sweeteners

Another harmful substance that you will want to eliminate from your diet is artificial sweeteners. Aspartame and saccharin are some of the most toxic compounds that have ever been added to our food supply. Although they are advertised as "low in calories" and a "healthy alternative to sugar," they are dangerous neurotoxins that trick a person's brain into thinking something is sweet when it's not.

Aspartame is comprised of three chemicals: aspartic acid (40%), phenylalanine (50%) and methanol (10%). Because aspartic acid is a neurotransmitter, it has the ability to facilitate the transmission of information from neuron to neuron. When aspartic acid and phenylalanine are introduced into a person's brain, they have the ability to excite brain cells, making that person think the food they're eating is sweet.

The only problem with tricking a person's brain into thinking something is sweet when it's really not is that aspartic acid and phenylalanine have the ability to overstimulate and excite brain cells to death.[2]

When too many brain cells die from being overexcited, that person may experience the following warning signs: headaches, dizziness, seizures, nausea, muscle spasms, weight gain, depression, fatigue, irritability, insomnia, vision problems, loss of hearing, anxiety, vertigo and memory loss. Because the prolonged use of artificial sweeteners can cause permanent brain damage, the following mental disorders may result: brain tumors, multiple sclerosis, epilepsy, chronic fatigue syndrome, Alzheimer's and Parkinson's disease.

The other ingredient found in aspartame is methanol, which is commonly referred to as wood alcohol. In its natural form, methanol is a deadly poison. When methanol is broken down and absorbed in the body, it turns into formaldehyde. Symptoms of methanol poisoning include headaches, ear buzzing, dizziness, nausea, vertigo, memory lapses, blurry vision, retinal damage, blindness and behavioral disturbances.

Overcoming Food Addictions

The first step in overcoming a food addiction would be to turn to God in prayer and ask for assistance. In the same way that Adam and Eve could commune with God during the time of the evening breeze, so too can you ask for all your needs. We have a loving Heavenly Father who knows every detail of our lives, and he desperately wants to help us overcome all our problems and difficulties. Because God will never violate anyone's free will, the first step in breaking free would be to start with a simple prayer:

Dear Heavenly Father, please forgive me for turning to food as a source of comfort. I turn away from all fleeting pleasures and invite your presence into my life and heart. Please transform my life and remove all worry, fear and anxiety from me. I desire to enter into a deeper and more meaningful relationship with you. I want to feel your loving embrace. Please remove all food cravings from me, restore my neurological pathways and rebalance my brain chemistry. I want to be the kind of person that you have created me to be.

After you have asked God for assistance, the next step would be to resist the temptations whenever they occur. According to Matthew 4:3–4, Jesus was also tempted by food. After Jesus had fasted 40 days and nights in the wilderness, he was famished. *The tempter came and said to him, "If you are the Son of God, command these stones to become loaves of bread." But he answered, "It is written, 'One does not live by bread alone, but by every word that comes from the mouth of God.'"*

In the same way that Jesus resisted the devil's temptation by quoting Scripture, you can also rebuke your own temptations by quoting passages from God's Word. For example, the next time you feel tempted to buy ice cream, address the temptation directly by saying, *One does not live by sweets alone but by every word that comes from the mouth of God.* Another option would be to personalize a quote from Ephesians 5:18, which says, *Do not get drunk with wine, for that is debauchery; but be filled with the Spirit.* Instead of using wine as an example of debauchery, just replace the word "wine" with any other temptation that you may be facing.

If you find yourself being tempted to buy a candy bar at the gas station or find yourself being tempted by the vending machines at work, it may be helpful to ask for the full armor of God. The full armor is described in Ephesians 6:10–17 as follows: *Finally, be strong in the Lord and in the strength of his power. Put on the whole armor of God, so that you may be able to stand against the wiles of the devil.*

For our struggle is not against enemies of blood and flesh, but against the rulers, against the authorities, against the cosmic powers of this present darkness, against the spiritual forces of evil in the heavenly places. Therefore take up the whole armor of God, so that you may be able to withstand on that evil day, and having done everything, to stand firm.

Stand therefore, and fasten the belt of truth around your waist, and put on the breastplate of righteousness. As shoes for your feet put on whatever will make you ready to proclaim the gospel of peace. With all of these, take the shield of faith, with which you will be able to quench all the flaming arrows of the evil one. Take the helmet of salvation, and the sword of the Spirit, which is the word of God.

After you have identified the source of your temptation, it will be easier to pray against that situation in the future. If the vending machines at work are the problem, simply ask God to give you more spiritual strength:

Dear Heavenly Father, I come before you in great need of your assistance. Please give me the spiritual strength I need to resist every form of temptation. Please fasten the belt of truth and discipline around my waste and give me a newfound respect for my body. Please bestow upon me your full armor and place your protective barrier between me and the vending machines. May the sword of the Spirit—the Word of God—be constantly on my lips as I expose every lie of the enemy.

After you have prayed against the source of the temptation, the next step would be to deal with any underlying personal, emotional or spiritual issues. Usually when most people overeat, there's a deeper conflict of worry, fear or anxiety that has been troubling their hearts. In these circumstances, a person's quiet time with the Lord (or daily devotionals) may have slowly diminished to the point of nonexistence.

Instead of dealing with the uncomfortable feelings deep within our hearts, it's much easier to stimulate the pleasure centers of our brains with an excessive amount of salt, fat and sweets. When this occurs, it will be necessary to turn back to God with our full devotion so that the Lord can help us work through any underlying issues.

By working in partnership with God, you will be able to overcome all temptations and live in harmony with every aspect of his creation.

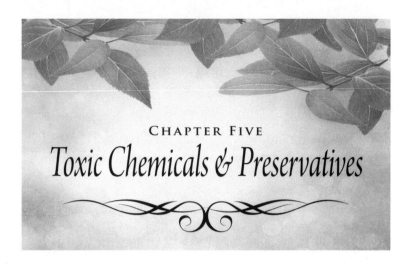

CHAPTER FIVE

Toxic Chemicals & Preservatives

One day when Adam and Eve were working in the field next to their home, the Lord stopped by to visit his beloved children. As the Lord approached from the distance, Adam ran to meet him, saying, "You won't believe what happened. One of your banana trees malfunctioned."

"How is that possible?" God asked.

"I followed all your instructions," Adam said. "After harvesting the fruit, I cut down the primary stalk so the secondary shoot could produce; but for some reason, the fruit tastes terrible."

"Let's examine the fruit more closely," God said.

"Please come and see," Eve said. "It's over here."

As Adam and Eve approached the decomposing pile of bananas, God said, "Do you see the square edges, how the fruit didn't have a chance to fully develop into a rounded and robust shape?"

"But I thought it was okay to harvest green bananas,"

Adam said. "In the past, they always turned yellow and became sweet. Besides, if you wait too long, the fruit bats and monkeys take everything."

"I understand how the fruit was harvested too early," Eve said. "But why did the bananas start to decompose?"

"And why do they taste terrible?" Adam asked.

"Because the bananas were harvested too early, the starches and acids started to break down, creating an altered chemical composition, which in turn caused the unpleasant taste. Because the fruit could no longer protect itself, different species of fungus started consuming the nutrients."

"That's very interesting," Eve said.

"If you leave the bananas sitting on the ground like that, larger detritivores will soon assimilate the nutrients back into the soil," God said.

"What's a detritivore?" Adam asked.

"They're an important part of my creation," God said. "When a leaf falls to the ground, a microscopic army of fungus and bacteria will start breaking down the organic matter. If plants and animals never decayed after death, the face of the earth would be covered with their remains. Larger detritivores, including vultures, seagulls, slugs, snails and even earthworms, assist in this process. Whenever you see mushrooms growing on the forest floor, know that there's a colony of fungus beneath the soil recycling the nutrients."

"So that's why we shouldn't eat mushrooms," Eve

said. "But is there a way to extend the life of bananas after harvesting?"

"It's best to consume your food directly from the garden," God said. "Any time you extend the life of food, it degrades the food's nutritional value. Remember, there's a time and season for every matter under heaven—a time for planting and a time for harvesting. It's not possible to extend the life of food without experiencing the natural consequences."

Because Adam and Eve continued asking God for a way to extend the life of their food, God showed his beloved children how to make raisins. The process is very simple. All you need to do is separate the grapes from the vine and leave them in the hot sun for five days. After the water evaporates, the enzymes and phytonutrients will die, but you will be able to preserve the sweet sugary content of the grapes for an extended period of time.

Another way to extend the life of food comes from the modern-day method of home canning. This process works by removing the majority of oxygen from glass containers, because without an adequate oxygen supply, mold cannot grow. For example, when canning applesauce, the fruit is usually cut up and cooked. The warm applesauce is then placed inside heated glass jars, causing the contents to expand.

After airtight lids are placed on the jars and left to cool, the applesauce contracts, causing a vacuum and a decreased percentage of oxygen inside the sealed container. Although it's possible to preserve the sugar content of apples (and some of their flavor) for an extended period of time, the heat and cooking process will destroy the apples' natural vitamins, phytonutrients and enzymes.

Food Preservatives

In our modern-day food processing industry, dried fruit is preserved using sulfites. Although sulfites are effective at preventing mold and discoloration, they can also make a person sick. The United States Food and Drug Administration estimates that more than a million people are allergic to sulfites, causing a range of mild to severe reactions, including difficulty breathing, headaches, skin irritations, abdominal pain and anaphylactic shock.[1] Sulfites are also used as a bleaching agent, and they destroy vitamins. Sulfites are commonly used in canned olives, condiments, dehydrated potatoes, molasses and baked goods.

Another dangerous preservative that our food processing industry uses is sodium nitrate. Although this preservative prevents bacterial growth in processed meat products, according to the United States Environmental Protection Agency, the consumption of nitrates increases a person's risk of cancer, leukemia and brain tumors.[2] Although sodium nitrate may sound like another form of salt, it's actually highly carcinogenic once it enters the human digestive system and can wreak havoc on a number of internal organs.

Sodium nitrates are preferred by the food processing industry because they can transform brown, dead-looking meat into fresh-looking, bright-red products. Sodium nitrates are used in bacon, ham, hot dogs, sausage, corned beef, smoked fish and other processed meats.

Dangerous Food Additives

In addition to using harmful chemicals to extend the expiration date of our groceries, the food processing industry also uses thickeners, emulsifiers and other synthetic compounds that are never truly disclosed on the product's label, except under the term *natural flavors.*

A good example of a dangerous food additive that acts as a thickening agent and emulsifier is called *carrageenan* or *xanthan gum.* These additives can be found in a wide variety of products, including soy and almond milk. Although most people consider almond milk a healthy alternative to dairy products, the problem is that almonds don't contain any milk. To solve this problem, food chemists would need to take ground almond powder and convert it into a thick, creamy, delicious beverage.

> **Ingredients for Almond Beverage**
>
> Filtered water, almonds, tricalcium phosphate, sea salt, gellan gum, dipotassium phosphate, xanthan gum, natural flavors, sunflower lecithin, vitamin A palmitate, vitamin D_2, dl-alpha tocopherol acetate.

In order to understand the challenge that food chemists face, it may be helpful to make your own almond milk. All you need to do is grind up some almonds and place the powder in water. There are only two healthy ingredients that your body needs, almonds and water, but because the general public would never purchase clear water with almond powder that has settled on the bottom of the container, food chemists would need to add thickening agents such as carrageenan and xanthan gum.

To solve this problem, food chemists looked to

nature and discovered pond scum floating on the surface of the water. Because the pond scum could float on the surface, was layered throughout the mid-section and could thrive at the bottom, it acted as the perfect thickening agent. The only problem was that the pond scum is green (or red) and needed to be bleached with industrial solvents.

In an attempt to manufacture the perfect thickening agent, a bacteria called *xanthomonas campestris* was placed in a growth medium containing sugars and other industrial waste products. Once the bacteria spread throughout the pool, an indigestible polysaccharide was harvested, purified, dried and ground into powder to be sold as xanthan gum. Carrageenan has a similar manufacturing process, except it's extracted from red algae.

After the invention of thickening agents, food chemists were able to mix water with ground almond powder, and after adding carrageenan or xanthan gum, the indigestible polysaccharides acted as the perfect thickening agent. It bound all the ingredients together. The substance floated on the top of the container, emulsified the mid-section and settled at the bottom. It turned ordinary water (with almond powder) into a thick, creamy beverage. The other additional ingredients necessary to sell the product to the public was sugar and salt to make it taste better, food coloring to turn the fluid white, and preservatives to prevent the pond scum from coming back to life.

Although carrageenan and xanthan gum are found in a wide variety of so-called "natural health products," according to studies conducted by the World Health Organization's International Agency for Research on

Cancer, carrageenan is a known carcinogen—a substance that causes colon cancer in laboratory animals.[3]

Because there are only two ingredients in almond milk that your body needs (almonds and water), you would be better off buying a bag of raw almonds and drinking pure water. As for the rest of the ingredients: *tricalcium phosphate* is used as a thickening agent and to add opacity. Tricalcium phosphate is also used to make baby powder.

> ### Ingredients for Almond Milk
>
> Filtered water, almonds, evaporated cane juice, calcium carbonate, sea salt, potassium citrate, carrageenan, sunflower lecithin, vitamin A palmitate, vitamin D2, d-alpha-tocopherol.

Calcium carbonate is used to add a white color and also used in paint manufacturing to provide a thick white base to latex paints. It's almost impossible to find out what food chemists hide in natural flavors. *Dl-alpha tocopherol acetate* is a synthetic version of vitamin E. Because carrageenan and xanthan gum are both indigestible substances, they can also contribute to acid reflux, bloating, indigestion and irritable bowel syndrome.

Synthetic & Natural Flavors

A good example of how processed food manufacturers are able to hide any kind of ingredient they want under the term "natural flavors" comes from Coca-Cola. The ingredients listed on a regular can of Coke include "carbonated water, high fructose corn syrup, caramel color, phosphoric acid, natural flavors and caffeine."[4]

Coca-Cola was created in 1886 by an Atlanta pharmacist named John Pemberton, who modeled the beverage after a popular French coca-leaf extract wine. To avoid liquor regulations in the United States, Pemberton mixed his coca-leaf extract formula with sweet syrup instead of alcohol. He also added kola-nut extract, giving the product its trade name Coca-Cola.

When cocaine became illegal in the United States during 1914, a public debate arose over the company's use of the coca-leaf extract along with the product's potential for containing alkaloid compounds similar to cocaine. At the time, the company's founders defended the use of cocaine, citing the drug's medicinal benefits. Although company executives cut back on the use of cocaine to a "mere trace" in 1914, Coca-Cola wouldn't become completely cocaine-free until 1929, when scientists perfected the process of removing all psychoactive elements from the coca-leaf extract.[5]

Today the recipe for Coca-Cola is a highly prized company secret. Only a few people in the world are reported to know the exact ingredients. The company has even built an elaborate tourist attraction in Atlanta, Georgia, including a large vault (with red carpeting) that supposedly protects the secret content of Coca-Cola's natural flavors.[6]

Another ingredient found in Coca-Cola is phosphoric acid. In its pure form, phosphoric acid is a colorless and odorless crystal made several different ways. One manufacturing process involves stripping phosphate rocks with sulfuric acid. The other thermal process involves spraying phosphorus into a furnace where it is burnt at over 3,000 degrees.

Phosphoric acid is commercially used in fertilizers, polishes and dyes. It's added to soft drinks to provide a sharper, tangy taste. It also slows down the growth of mold and bacteria in sugary products. Phosphoric acid is also found in sports drinks, bottled teas, fruit-flavored beverages, cottage cheese, breakfast bars and processed meats.

Another ingredient found in Coca-Cola (and many other processed foods) is caramel coloring. Although the name may sound safe enough, as if it were comprised of ordinary caramel or caramel candy—the kind you could make at home by melting sugar in a saucepan—far from being safe, this artificial brown coloring is made by reacting sugars with ammonia and sulfites under high pressure and temperatures.

During this manufacturing process, two toxins are formed, 2-methylimidazole and 4-methylimidazole, which in government-conducted studies, caused leukemia, lung, liver or thyroid cancer in laboratory animals. According to the National Toxicology Program, a division of the National Institute of Environmental Health Sciences, there is "clear evidence" that both 2-MI and 4-MI are animal carcinogens.[7] Processed foods that contain caramel coloring include soy sauce, dark beer, chocolate, dark breads, gravies, soups and sauces.

Chemically Engineered Scents

Because our sense of smell makes up 80 percent of our sense of taste, food engineers have been creating mixtures of chemicals similar to those found in perfume. The goal of a successful food engineer is to create a flavor (or a sense of smell) that tastes better than natural foods. They work extremely hard at creating chemical compositions to give their customers a fresh, mouthwatering taste sensation so that the highly processed foods they work on can sit on the shelf for more than a year and still taste delicious.

A good example of how natural flavors are used comes from store-bought orange juice. After the oranges have been processed with a mechanical press to extract all the juices, the solution needs to be pasteurized to kill any bacteria that may be present. When orange juice is pasteurized with heat, most of the natural flavors are burnt off in the process, leaving behind a stale, flat-tasting product. In order to make pasteurized orange juice taste like it's fresh, flavor engineers create chemical scents to give the juice a specific taste and smell, which makes the consumer think the juice is fresh.

Flavor engineers also want to create a taste sensation that's short-lived so that the consumer uses more of the manufacturer's product. They want to create a wonderful burst of flavor in the beginning, but if the taste lingers too long, the consumer may stop eating, so the taste needs to be short-lived so that the consumer falls in love with the product and develops a craving for more.

According to the United States Food and Drug Administration, the only difference between natural and artificial flavoring is the origin of the chemicals. When asked to define the term *natural*, the FDA responded with a statement saying, "It is difficult to define a food product that is 'natural' because the food has probably been processed and is no longer the product of the earth."[8] Although foods with *natural flavors* listed on the package may sound safer, the actual chemical structure of the ingredients can be exactly the same as those of *artificial flavors*.

Toxic Chemicals Cause Cancer

Consuming an unhealthy diet of toxic chemicals and preservatives is dangerous, because when given enough time, these deadly chemicals have the ability to overwhelm a person's liver and end up being stored inside their fat cells. Once a cell's ability to read its own DNA has been compromised, the cell can mutate, take on a life of its own and migrate to other parts of the body in the form of cancer. A good example of how processed foods have the ability to cause cancer comes from a young man named Luke who was diagnosed with stage-3 colon cancer.

Although Luke appeared to be strong and healthy, he continued to consume an unhealthy diet of commercially processed foods for many years. Because Luke didn't smoke or drink alcohol, he figured that he could eat anything he wanted. Then one day, he began to experience sharp abdominal pains. To make matters worse, Luke also worked in a high-stress environment and wasn't getting enough sleep at night.

Eventually Luke went to see his doctor because he wasn't feeling well. After performing several tests, Luke's doctor diagnosed him with stage-3 colon cancer. Because there was a golf ball-sized tumor growing in Luke's abdomen and four of his lymph nodes tested positive for adenocarcinoma, the surgeon performed an operation and removed 18 inches of his colon. After the operation, the doctors wanted to administer 12 months of chemotherapy.

The reason that Luke's oncologist wanted to administer chemotherapy was because the cancer could always "come back" and spread to other parts of his body. That's because cancer is a systemic disease affecting the entire body. The surgery that removed Luke's colon was never designed to cure cancer. Because Luke's doctor knew there were circulating tumor cells and circulating stem cells in other parts of his body, he wanted to start chemotherapy treatment immediately.

Because Luke knew that chemotherapy was a toxic poison that could cause permanent damage to his brain, nerves, heart, lungs, liver, kidneys and bladder, he became very hesitant to receive the treatment and began to pray, "Dear God, if there's a better way, please show me." Meanwhile, Luke's doctor became even more insistent and told Luke, "You're crazy if you don't accept my treatment plan."

The idea of poisoning his way back to health didn't make sense to Luke. He knew that chemotherapy would destroy his immune system and make the cancer stem cells even more aggressive. Given the fact that chemotherapy had an exaggerated success rate by the medical community, Luke decided to heal his body by utilizing an all-natural approach. He started the process by reading a book entitled, *God's Way To Ultimate Health*.

During this time, Luke purchased a high-quality juicer and a distiller to purify his drinking water. Then he started fasting. Luke would drink eight (eight-ounce) servings of organic carrot, celery, beet and ginger juices throughout the day. When he wasn't fasting, Luke would eat an organic green apple or grapefruit in the morning, an organic salad for lunch, another salad for dinner, and in-between, he would snack on healthy nuts and coconut berry smoothies throughout the day.

Luke continued with his customized fasting routine for 90 days and eventually added a little animal protein back into his diet. Since that time, Luke has been cancer free. He is currently living on an 80-percent raw vegetarian diet and can say with confidence that his body has the ability to heal itself of cancer. Luke would never go back to eating processed foods again because of his newfound health, strength and energy that he is now experiencing with an all-natural diet.

Giving an Account before God

Maybe the most important reason to stop consuming commercially processed foods is to give an account before God regarding everything you eat during the day. When a man purchases organic fruits, vegetables, grains and seeds with a little bit of organic animal protein, he knows exactly where those products came from and exactly what's in everything he eats. It's not possible to give an account before God when you consume commercially processed foods, because there are thousands of man-made chemicals in our modern-day food supply that are hidden on the label under misleading terms.

A good example of a food additive that you will *not* want to put into your body is L-cysteine. It's a nonessential amino acid that is currently being added to baked goods as a "dough conditioner." While some L-cysteine is created in laboratories, most of it is extracted from cheap and abundant protein sources, including human hair, chicken feathers and petroleum by-products.

Most of the human hair used to make L-cysteine is swept up off the floors of barbershops and hair salons from China. After the human hair and duck feathers have been dissolved in acid, the L-cysteine is isolated through a chemical process, packaged and shipped off to commercial bakers in the United States.[9]

Because it is unfathomable that commercial bakers would use L-cysteine that has been sourced from duck feathers and human hair, you may want to conduct your own Internet research using the key words "Source of L-cysteine" to see for yourself. While you're at it, you may want to research two other toxic chemicals used as "dough conditioners," including ammonium sulfate and potassium bromate.

Even though potassium bromate has been banned in Canada, Europe and China, it's still available in the United States and being added to our baked goods under the appearance of "enriched flour." In the event that you cannot give an account before God for the reasons why you have been consuming Chinese human hair in your baked goods, you may want to consider making your own bread.

The following bread recipe is simple and fun to make. It turns out perfect every time. The best part about making your own bread is being able to give an account before God concerning every ingredient that you consume during the day. This bread recipe contains four simple ingredients: water, flour, yeast and salt. The salt is optional.

Fast & Easy Bread Recipe

Standard
3 cups white flour
3/8 teaspoon instant yeast
1/2 teaspoon salt
1 1/2 cups water

Whole Wheat
2 cups white flour
1 cup whole wheat flour
3/8 teaspoon instant yeast
1/2 teaspoon salt
1 9/16 cups water

Total Whole Wheat
3 cups whole wheat flour
1/2 teaspoon instant yeast
1/2 teaspoon salt
1 2/3 cups water

Quick Rise
3 cups white unbleached flour
3/4 teaspoon (rapid rise) yeast
1/2 teaspoon salt
1 1/2 cups warm water
Let stand seven hours, plus one
hour before baking.

Instructions

Combine flour, yeast and salt (along with optional ingredients) in a large bowl. Add water until blended. Cover bowl with loose-fitting lid (or plastic wrap) and set aside for 12 to 18 hours. Overnight works great. Two hours before baking, turn the dough over on itself by running a large spoon around the perimeter of the bowl several times. Preheat a cast-iron pot (or casserole dish with glass lid) in the oven at 450 degrees for at least 15 minutes before cooking. Pour (or roll out) the bread dough into the preheated pot and bake 30 minutes with the lid on. Then remove the lid and bake an additional 12 to 16 minutes. (Use the longer 16-minute cooking time for higher elevations.) Remove bread from oven and place on rack to cool.

Raisin & Cinnamon Bread

Make the standard bread recipe and add ¾ cup raisins along with 1 teaspoon cinnamon.

Oatmeal or Buckwheat Bread

Make the standard recipe and add ¾ cup (presoaked and drained) rolled oats or buckwheat. When adding additional ingredients, you will want to keep the moisture in the dough consistent with the standard recipe.

Additional Options

Try adding olives, cranberries and pecans, or different combinations of flour, or even powdered milk for protein. When adding an apple, place the fruit in a blender with a little water. Then use the blended sauce as part of your liquid measurement. When adding ingredients that will make the dough sticky (like blended fruit), you may want to coat the outside of the dough with flour two hours before baking.

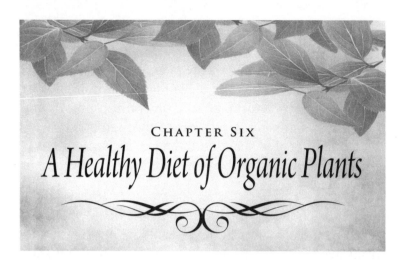

CHAPTER SIX

A Healthy Diet of Organic Plants

After God created the heavens and earth he said, *"Let the earth put forth vegetation: plants yielding seed, and fruit trees of every kind on earth that bear fruit with the seed in it." And it was so. The earth brought forth vegetation: plants yielding seed of every kind, and trees of every kind bearing fruit with the seed in it. And God saw that it was good. ~ Genesis 1:11–12*

To understand how God created over several hundred thousand species of plants in one day, it might be helpful to picture a giant ladder towering a mile high. God formed the ladder out of deoxyribonucleic acid (DNA) and twisted the structure to give it a double helix design so that it looked like a spiraling staircase. Next, God filled in parts of the ladder with genes to give each element of his creation different characteristics.

For example, the first hundred steps of the ladder allowed a plant to sense its environment and grow in the direction of the sunlight. The next hundred steps of the ladder controlled how fast the plant could grow. After God filled all the rungs of the ladder with thousands of genes, he studied the genetic blueprint to make sure nothing was missing. God worked through every possible design detail to make sure the genetic structure was complete and filled with everything the plant needed to sustain life.

The genetic information contained in a plant's DNA would also need to provide all the information the plant needed to create seeds, defend itself from invasive species, put forth flowers, produce sweet-smelling nectar, repair damaged branches and produce fruit. After God finished loading the ladder with everything the plant needed for life, he reduced the ladder down in size so small that it would fit inside the cell's nucleus.

After placing a copy of the plant's genetic blueprint inside every cell in the plant, God spoke life unto the plant and it became a living organism. God was so happy with the genetic blueprint that he created several hundred thousand more species of plants. When it came time to create humanity, God used the same chemical building blocks of DNA—a phosphate ladder filled with adenine, cytosine, guanine and thymine—to bring Adam and Eve's bodies to life.

Although humans have more chromosomes than plants, many plants have more genes than humans. For example, it's estimated that the human body contains 22,000 different sets of genes, while a grapevine has 30,000 different genes that allow it to flourish in different climates. A raspberry has a smaller genetic blueprint (or genome) than humans, but an onion has 12 times that amount.

Another incredible design feature of plants is their ability to use photoreceptors to perceive light. For example, a vine can sense a nearby light source and grow in that direction. Plants also have the ability to measure changes in the quality of light that's being reflected from the leaves of adjacent plants. Plants also use chemical sensors to gauge their proximity to other plants, and when necessary, respond accordingly by changing their growth patterns.

Plants also have the ability to produce their own energy. The process is called *photosynthesis* and works through a series of chemical reactions where a plant converts carbon dioxide and water into sugar that it uses for fuel. The by-product of photosynthesis is oxygen, which we need to breathe. Not only can plants make their own food and provide humans with oxygen, but plants are the only food source on earth that sustain all other forms of life.

Plants also have the ability to take inorganic minerals from the ground and convert them into the organic minerals that our bodies need. For example, the human body needs a small amount of magnesium, potassium and calcium every day to build healthy bones. Although these minerals are found in rocks, it's not possible to grind up rocks and, after eating the powder, expect the human body to effectively utilize those minerals. In order for the human body to utilize the minerals found in rocks, a plant needs to convert the inorganic minerals into organic minerals. Once the plant completes the conversion process, we can then consume the plant and effectively absorb those minerals into our bodies.

Genetically Modified Organisms

Although plants have been designed by God to provide humanity with life, health, healing, oxygen and valuable nutrients from the soil, it didn't take long before scientists started interfering with God's creation. A good example of how genetic engineers have been trying to alter humanity's food source comes from a company called *Monsanto*.

In the past, Monsanto has been responsible for inventing some of the world's most controversial products, including Agent Orange, Saccharin and PCBs. Today, the biotech giant produces a herbicide called *Roundup* along with seeds whose genes have been genetically modified to survive Roundup's plant-killing ingredient, glyphosate.[1]

In the past, plants were genetically modified using a gene gun, which shot metal particles coated with foreign DNA into a plant's tissue. A more advanced method of inserting genes into a plant's DNA involves Monsanto's Trojan horse approach. In this process, seedlings are heated up to place the plants under stress, making them more susceptible to a pathogen called *agrobacterium*.

To create "Roundup Ready" plants, scientists from Monsanto identified a particular strain of agrobacterium that was not affected by glyphosate (the active ingredient in Roundup), so they inserted the gene into the chromosomes of soybeans. Because the plant survived and was able to produce seeds that carried the same genetic traits, they were able to create the world's first Roundup Ready food source.[2]

Roundup Ready soybeans were brought to the market in 1996, followed by alfalfa, corn, cotton, sugar beets and canola. Today, more than 90 percent of our nation's soybeans and 70 percent of our nation's corn use genetically modified seeds. Farmers are able to plant Roundup Ready seeds, spray their crops with glyphosate and within a few days, all the weeds will die while their genetically modified plants will continue growing to maturity.

The active ingredient in Roundup kills plants by preventing them from forming three necessary amino acids: tryptophan, phenylalanine and tyrosine. One of the major problems with spraying crops with glyphosate is that the chemical becomes absorbed into the plant and cannot be washed off. Studies have found residue from glyphosate remaining stable inside produce for more than a year, even after the produce has been commercially processed. Glyphosate has also been found in the tissue and organs of cows that consume glyphosate-treated alfalfa, corn and soy.

Another problem with spraying millions of gallons of glyphosate on American soil every year is that it acts as a chelating agent, forming chemical bonds with the minerals in the ground and inside the plants. When glyphosate forms a chemical bond with essential minerals in plants (calcium, zinc and manganese), it immobilizes the plant's ability to utilize those minerals, making them unavailable for our bodies to use when we consume the plant.

Currently there are more than 180 genetically modified crops approved for use in the United States, including two types of apples—Arctic Golden Delicious and Arctic Granny Smith. There are 20 different options for farmers who want to plant genetically modified canola, 28 options for genetically modified cotton and 40 different types of genetically modified corn.[3]

Other genetically modified crops include two options for melons, three versions of papayas and 40 different kinds of potatoes, including New Leaf Plus Russet Burbank Potatoes. There's also rice, 24 varieties of soybeans, squash, sugar beets, sugarcane, eight different varieties of tomatoes, and don't forget the wheat. There's even a genetically engineered version of salmon available called *AquAdvantage* that has been approved by the United States Food and Drug Administration.[4]

Another danger in consuming genetically modified plants is that many varieties have been engineered to produce their own pesticides. Several varieties of corn have been modified so that the plant produces a chemical substance that is toxic to insect larvae. The primary concern with eating corn that has been genetically modified to produce its own pesticide is that when eating the corn, a person would also be consuming the toxic pesticide that the plant produces.

A Swiss biotech company called *Syngenta* is also working to create a genetically modified version of golden rice that contains higher concentrations of vitamin A. Although this may sound like a good idea, it's not necessary because organic fruits and vegetables naturally contain more vitamins and minerals than their commercially produced counterparts.

Organic fruits and vegetables also taste better. They are free of dangerous herbicides, pesticides, fungicides and fertilizers. When you purchase an organic tomato, you can rest assured that it has not been inserted into a gas-ripening chamber. By choosing organic meats and dairy products, you will decrease your exposure to dangerous antibiotics, toxic chemicals and synthetic hormones.

The Healing Power of Organic Plants

Consuming a healthy diet of organic fruits, vegetables, grains and seeds will also strengthen and support your body's ability to heal itself. A good example of how the human body can heal itself through an all-natural diet of organic produce comes from a woman named Janelle who was diagnosed with stage-3 breast cancer.

When Janelle went to see her doctor, she was informed that she only had six months to live. The medical staff at the hospital offered her chemotherapy and radiation, saying, "It will make you very sick, but if you're lucky, it will increase your chances for survival."

Janelle listened very carefully to everything the medical professionals recommended, but after conducting her own research on the history of chemotherapy, she began to question the wisdom of putting any more toxic chemicals inside her body. She kept asking herself, "If my body has already been compromised, why would I want to harm it even further with radiation and chemotherapy?"

After conducting her own research, Janelle discovered that chemotherapy was originally used on the battlefields of Belgium during the first World War. According to reports, the soldiers noticed a strange peppery smell in the air and they soon began to itch uncontrollably. Within a few days, the soldiers started coughing up blood and developed horrific blisters and sores. They had been poisoned by mustard gas, one of the most deadly chemical weapons deployed in battle. Fully clothed soldiers wearing gas masks were left defenseless, because the toxin could be absorbed through their skin.

In an attempt to discover an antidote for mustard gas, a team of researchers discovered that the victims had a surprisingly low number of immune cells in their blood. This made the researchers think that if mustard gas could destroy normal white blood cells, it seemed likely that it could also destroy cancerous cells.

After conducting successful animal trials, the researchers started looking for a volunteer to use mustard gas on as a form of cancer treatment. They found a patient with advanced lymphoma who had a massive tumor. After administering a number of treatments with a compound that was used to make mustard gas, the man started showing signs of improvement.

At first he began sleeping better at night and then he started feeling better. It was a monumental moment in the history of modern-day medicine and the beginning of chemotherapy. Although the mustard gas was able to kill the man's cancer cells, it also killed many other cells in the man's body, and unfortunately, he died six months later.

As Janelle continued contemplating the history and origins of chemotherapy, she kept asking herself, "If I only have six months to live, why would I want to endure a poisonous treatment that will harm my body in hopes of extending my life another six months? It just doesn't make sense. Because my body is obviously in trouble, doesn't it make more sense to help my body heal with the nutrients it needs?"

Instead of receiving her doctor's poisonous treatment plan, Janelle began reading several health and healing books on cancer and decided to try a 42-day fast as described in *The Breuss Cancer Cure*. The book outlined different forms of fasting for different types of cancer. According to its recommended treatment plan for breast cancer, Janelle's 42-day fast would consist mostly of beetroot, Brussels sprouts, broccoli, cabbage and wheatgrass.

Her goal was to starve the cancer cells to death and keep her body alive by drinking the minimal amount of highly nutritious juice. The benefit of a 42-day fast was that when her body was being starved for fuel, it would start consuming all of her fat cells and all other nonessential tissues, including all her cancer cells and tumors. Although Janelle received many warnings that the 42-day fast would make her very weak and tired, she actually found she had more energy.

During this time, Janelle started increasing the amount of oxygen that her body was receiving. Because cancer cells cannot survive in an oxygen-rich environment, Janelle started increasing her oxygen intake by running and spending time in nature. Being surrounded by green plants and clean air made her feel more at peace. She also focused on her breathing techniques, making sure she took deeper, fuller, more relaxed breaths of air.

Janelle also fought the cancer from a spiritual perspective by eliminating all forms of stress and negative emotions from her life. When she allowed her negative thoughts to run wild with fear and worry, her body would release powerful hormones that produced acidity and suppressed her immune system. Janelle fought these temptations with prayer, quiet time and being alone with God, surrounded by nature.

After the 42-day fast came to a completion, Janelle continued juicing and started eating an all-raw, vegetarian diet. She didn't want to cook her foods any longer because cooking kills enzymes, and without her food's natural enzymes, her body wouldn't be able to absorb the maximum amount of nutrients that she needed. By consuming an all-raw diet, the molecular structure of her food would remain intact, allowing her body to receive more vitamins and minerals.

As Janelle continued to enjoy a healthy, all-raw, natural diet of organic fruits, vegetables, grains and seeds, her body healed itself. Today Janelle is cancer free, she continues to run and looks younger, stronger and healthier than she did 20 years ago.

Beginning the Journey

To begin the journey back to the Garden of Eden, it will be helpful to remove all the commercially processed foods from your home. One option is to box up all the canned, prepackaged and processed foods and donate them to your local homeless shelter or food bank. The other option would be to bring a large trash can into your kitchen and start throwing away all the opened containers of condiments, snack crackers, chips, cookies, ice cream and everything else that contains salt, fat, sweets or preservatives.

Once you have completely cleared out all the toxic junk food from your house, you will need to restock your countertops, cupboards and refrigerator with healthy, organic foods that will bring health to your body and energy to your life. To begin this process, you may want to acquire a lot of fruit. Fruit is God's gift of sweetness and energy to humanity. Fruit is also loaded with digestive enzymes and cancer-fighting phytonutrients, vitamins and minerals.

Don't worry about consuming too many calories. Once you stop eating saturated animal fat, hydrogenated oil and man-made sweets, you will quickly lose a lot of weight and will need to eat a lot of fruit for energy. Some organic options to consider would include: apples, apricots, bananas, blueberries, cantaloupe, cranberries, grapefruit, grapes, kiwifruit, lemons, limes, oranges, papaya, pears, pineapple, plums, raspberries, strawberries and watermelon.

The next step after clearing out all the processed foods from your refrigerator would be to stock up on fresh organic vegetables. Some good places to shop would be at your local farmer's market and organic health food stores. Healthy organic produce options would include: asparagus, beets, bell peppers, bok choy, broccoli, Brussels sprouts, cabbage, carrots, cauliflower, celery, collard greens, cucumbers, eggplant, green beans, kale, leeks, mustard greens, olives, onions, sea vegetables, spinach, summer squash, sweet potatoes, swiss chard, tomatoes, turnip greens and winter squash.

For a good source of omega-3 and omega-6 fatty acids (the only fat your body needs), you may want to purchase the following nuts and seeds in their raw, natural state: almonds, chia, flaxseeds, pumpkin, sesame, sunflower and walnuts. Because flaxseeds will need to be ground before your body can utilize their valuable contents, you may want to purchase a seed or coffee grinder. Storing raw nuts, seeds and expeller-pressed oils inside the refrigerator will also help prevent oxidation.

Don't forget the importance of herbs and spices when restocking your kitchen. God has given us a wide variety of herbs and they all contain powerful phytonutrients to help your body stay young, strong and healthy. Fresh herbs are always better than dried because they're still alive. Some options to consider after pouring the contents of your salt shaker down the drain would be: basil, chili peppers, cilantro, cinnamon, cloves, cumin, dill, fennel, garlic, ginger, mustard, oregano, parsley, peppermint, rosemary, sage, thyme and turmeric.

Because whole grains are an important part of a healthy diet and a good source of fiber and protein, you may want to stock your cupboards with the following grains: amaranth, buckwheat, kamut, millet, oats, quinoa, teff and brown rice. In addition to whole grains, you may also want to purchase a wide variety of beans and legumes. They are high in fiber and a good source of protein. Your options for beans and legumes would include black, garbanzo, kidney, lima, navy, pinto and lentil.

Essential Amino Acids

There are 22 commonly known amino acids that are the basic building blocks for protein. Eight amino acids are considered essential because they need to be obtained from our food sources. A ninth amino acid (histidine) is considered essential only for infants. The other amino acids are considered nonessential because they can be manufactured within the human body. The essential amino acids your body needs are marked with an asterisk.

Alanine	Histidine	Pyrrolysine
Arginine	Isoleucine*	Selenocysteine
Asparagine	Leucine*	Serine
Aspartic acid	Lysine*	Taurine
Cysteine	Methionine*	Threonine*
Glutamic acid	Ornithine	Tryptophan*
Glutamine	Phenylalanine*	Tyrosine
Glycine	Proline	Valine*

Consuming a wide variety of whole, plant-based foods will provide all the essential amino acids your body needs for optimal growth, healing and health. For example, because most beans are low in methionine and high in lysine, it's best to mix them with rice, because rice is low in lysine and high in methionine. When you consume black beans and rice, your body is receiving all the essential amino acids it needs to build a complete form of protein.

Other examples of plant-based foods that contain all the essential amino acids include buckwheat, which is not a type of wheat at all, but rather a gluten-free relative of the rhubarb family. It's fast and easy to cook and contains 18 amino acids. One cup of uncooked grain contains 22.5 grams of protein. Quinoa also contains 18 amino acids and is a good source of iron, magnesium and manganese. One cup of uncooked quinoa contains 24 grams of protein.

A cup of chia seeds contains 18 amino acids with 35.2 grams of protein. Other plant-based foods that contain all the essential amino acids include carrots, celery, corn, cucumbers, broccoli, brown rice, green peppers, oats, pinto beans, potatoes and tomatoes.

Another amazing plant is wheatgrass. It contains 19 amino acids and will provide your body with 90 minerals. Wheatgrass is one of the best cancer-fighting foods on the planet and is considered *complete* because it can provide the human body with almost all of the nutrients it needs for energy and survival.

The only other item needed for your new life living in the Garden of Eden would be a small amount of organic animal protein. You may want to skip the animal protein for the first few months to see just how powerful a natural diet can be. One man named Thomas lost seven pounds the first week without even trying. A 60-year-old woman named Jill lost 55 pounds in her first year, and today she looks 20 years younger and has been blessed with fewer wrinkles and smoother skin.

Another man named Ted suffered from asthma, allergies and poor vision. Doctors blamed his condition on poor liver and kidney function, but after consuming an all-raw diet for nine months, all his symptoms completely disappeared. Another woman named Kathy was seeing several doctors and taking six different medications while her long list of medical problems kept growing. After embracing an all-raw, organic diet for six months, she was able to get off the medications, sleep through the night and has a newfound sense of love and excitement for life.

Custom Culinary Creations

Once you have completely removed all the junk food from your house and have loaded your countertops with fresh fruit, stocked your refrigerator with organic vegetables and purchased a wide variety of grains and legumes, the next step would be to get very creative. You will need to work out a custom culinary creation plan specifically designed to meet your own unique tastes and lifestyle.

To begin this process, all you need to do is go to your kitchen and start eating. It's possible to eat the vast majority of your vegetables raw. There's no need to watch cooking shows or to possess any kind of cooking skills. Just peel and eat. It's very simple. In the same way Adam and Eve walked through the Lord's garden and picked a cucumber, tomato and some kale, so too can you grab a handful of vegetables from your refrigerator and enjoy their natural goodness.

If you have an acorn, butternut or kabocha squash sitting on the counter, just cut a small cork-like hole in the side, and after removing the seeds, replace the cork and bake it in the oven for an hour. It would also be possible to include several sweet potatoes in the oven at the same time. To prepare some grains and legumes, all you need to do is soak them overnight and boil them the following morning for the least amount of time pos-sible—keeping in mind that cooking alters the chemical composition of your food and degrades its nutritional value.

When you are away from your home all day, it will be helpful to prepare an over-the-road salad in the morning and take it with you during the day. A nice over-the-road salad consists of a large container filled with tomatoes, asparagus, carrots, beets, summer squash or any other vegetable in your refrigerator.

There are only three simple rules to follow: limit salt, avoid fat and no sweets. You can add the fourth and fifth rules yourself—no processed foods or preservatives.

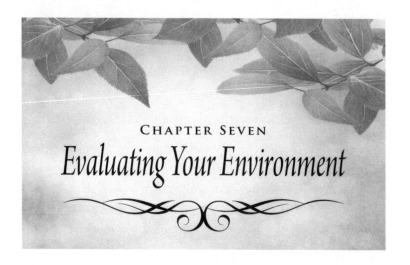

CHAPTER SEVEN

Evaluating Your Environment

It was a bright and beautiful morning in the garden. The sunrise had just emerged over the horizon, illuminating the sky with a soft reddish-orange glow amidst a thin layer of cirrocumulus clouds.

Adam was not feeling well, so God stopped by his beloved children's home for a visit. As the Lord approached from the distance, Eve ran to meet him, saying, "There's something wrong with Adam. Will you please help him?"

"That's why I have come," the Lord said.

Adam had been experiencing stomach cramps for several days, and he was resting inside his home. When he realized the Lord was outside, he rose to his feet and slowly walked over to meet him.

After greeting Adam the Lord said, "Think back and tell me when this discomfort first occurred."

"I don't know. Maybe a few days ago," Adam said.

"It started after he made friends with that miniature

horse," Eve said. "I know its been helping Adam do his work, but why does it have to live with us?"

"I like the donkey," Adam said. "He's my friend."

"I have given the donkey's digestive system hundreds of species of bacteria to help them break down cellulose when living in dry climates," God said. "Many species of those bacteria are present in the donkey's droppings."

"What does that mean?" Adam asked.

"When you look at the landscape, high upon the hillside where you have been keeping the donkey, do you see how it gently slopes down toward your water supply?"

"Ooo, it's the donkey's poo," Eve said.

"If you want, I will show you a natural spring where you may drink," God said. "They're easy to find, and there's one right over there."

As Adam and Eve walked with God into the forest behind their home, God began by saying, "It's best to wait for a dry period, when the heavens have withheld their rain. Then look along the lowest points for wet patches of soil. Once you find a trickle of water, follow it to its source. When you dig down, you will eventually find an impervious layer of rock."

"How does the water flow from a rock?" Adam asked.

"It flows upon the rock's surface beneath the soil," God said. "When the rain falls upon the mountains, a portion of water flows downstream while the rest seeps into the soil. The water that seeps into the soil slowly filters down through many layers of sandstone. Once the water hits an impervious layer of rock, it will follow the rock's surface until it reaches an opening in the ground."

"So the sandstone filters the water," Eve said, "making it pure."

"Very good, Eve," God said. "The water from the spring right over there is pure."

As Adam and Eve walked back to their home, the Lord began teaching his beloved children about the dangers that could occur to their future water supply once humanity began populating the face of the earth. One very serious danger that has occurred in our own lifetime comes from an oil and gas extraction process known as *hydraulic fracturing*.

When an oil company extracted natural gas in the past, they would drill a hole in the ground and allow the methane, propane and butane gases to rise to the surface. Then one day, a team of engineers discovered that if they pumped millions of gallons of water down one of the wells and placed the water under extremely high pressure, it had the ability to break apart rock formations and release even more gas.

To make this process more cost-effective, the team of engineers started adding hydrochloric acid to the water because it helped dissolve minerals and initiated more cracks in the rock. The engineers also wanted to pump silica sand into the cracks to keep the fractures open longer so that more gas would rise to the surface.

The problem with adding silica sand to the water was that the sand would sink to the bottom and didn't work very effectively, so the engineers began adding thickening agents to the water (petroleum distillate, methanol, guar gum, polysaccharide blend and ethylene glycol) to create a solution that would carry the sand into the cracks more efficiently.

The engineers also began adding friction reducers to make the sand flow more smoothly, and clay stabilizers (choline chloride, tetramethylammonium chloride, sodium chloride, isopropanol, methanol, formic acid and acetaldehyde), to prevent clay soils from swelling and shifting. After adding a few "corrosion inhibitors" to prevent the pipes from rusting and "pH-adjusting agents" (sodium hydroxide, potassium hydroxide, acetic acid, sodium carbonate and potassium carbonate), there are now hundreds of toxic chemicals being pumped into the ground at hydraulic fracturing sites.[1]

Although fracking fluids are pumped thousands of feet below the surface, methane gas and toxic chemicals have the ability to leach out of the fractured rock formations and contaminate the groundwater. Some of the known carcinogens that have poisoned the groundwater at hydraulic fracturing sites include uranium, mercury, lead, sulfuric acid, hydrochloric acid, BTEX compounds and formaldehyde.

Drinking Water Contamination

When public drinking water is tested at treatment facilities across the United States, hundreds of toxic chemicals turn up in the results. For example, Arizona, Idaho, Texas and New York have all recently reported finding uranium-238 in their public drinking water supplies. When drinking water from Pensacola, Florida, was tested, the following chemicals were detected: tetrachloroethylene, trichloroethylene, radium-226, radium-228, 1,2-dichloropropane and bromoform.[2]

In Las Vegas, Nevada, aluminum, molybdenum, arsenic and lead were found in the public water supply. Most of these dangerous toxins make their way into our drinking water through environmental contamination. For example, when a man's car overheats on the highway and his radiator hose bursts, several gallons of antifreeze will likely spill on the pavement. The next time it rains, the chemicals from the antifreeze, along with any motor oil stains on the road, will be washed into the storm sewer and eventually make their way into the soil.

As the earth becomes more populated, more toxic chemicals have been seeping through the soil, flowing downstream through underground waterways and contaminating public water supplies. To make matters worse, public water municipalities don't try to remove trace amounts of toxins from our drinking water, they only filter out large particles and add more chemicals. For example, chlorine is added to kill bacteria and fluorosilicic acid is added to prevent tooth decay.

Public Fluoride Program

The process of adding fluoride to the public water supply began in 1930 when a man discovered a group of people who had fewer cavities than the general population. After conducting more research, he discovered that the people with fewer cavities were also drinking natural spring water that contained fluoride. Because fluoride has the ability to harden tooth enamel, executives at a chemical manufacturing plant convinced public officials to add fluoride to the community water supply.

In 1945, the first community water fluoridation program was born, and since that time, the practice of adding fluoride to public drinking water has swept across the nation. According to the Centers for Disease Control and Prevention, approximately two-thirds of the population in America is currently receiving fluoride treatments in their water supply.[3] The CDC has plans to provide the remaining 100 million Americans with fluoridated water by the year 2020. Local water municipalities are allowed to use three chemicals to raise the fluoride levels in our drinking water, including sodium fluoride, sodium fluorosilicate and fluorosilicic acid.

Because fluorosilicic acid is also used for tanning animal hides, in glass production and as an impregnating agent to preserve wood and harden masonry, many health professionals are beginning to question the wisdom of adding fluorosilicic acid to drinking water. Because natural fluoride has the ability to harden tooth enamel, it would make more sense to add fluoride to toothpaste, and in the event that someone wanted more fluoride, there are many anti-cavity fluoride mouth-rinse products available in stores across the nation.

The only way to avoid the ever-increasing amount of toxic chemicals that have been seeping into our public drinking water is to buy a distiller. Although the typical charcoal water filters found in most homes are better than no form of protection, they are not effective at removing 99 percent of the contaminates. The typical charcoal filter will help absorb some of the chlorine that's added to drinking water along with a few large particles of sand and other debris, but it will never fully purify the water.

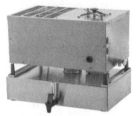

The only way to purify drinking water is by using a distiller. For less than $225, you can purchase a small countertop appliance that boils water inside a sealed chamber. As the water boils, steam rises to the top where it travels through cooling coils and condenses into a glass bottle. A high-quality, stainless-steel distiller that can produce eight gallons per day will cost around $800, but it will remove 100 percent of the toxins from your drinking water.

To give you an example of a distiller's effectiveness compared to a charcoal water filter, it's possible to run tap water through the average home water filtration unit all year long and never remove any solids. When you run five gallons of *filtered water* through a distiller, you will find solid mineral deposits building up on the inner walls of the tank and the water at the bottom of the tank will be heavily saturated.

Toxic Skin Absorption

After purchasing a high-quality distiller, the next step in evaluating your exposure to cancer-causing chemicals would be to examine everything you put on your skin. Because human skin is porous, it has the ability to absorb water along with many other chemicals. According to a study published in the *American Journal of Public Health,* 64 percent of the volatile carbon-based compounds found in public drinking water (toluene, ethylbenzene and styrene) could easily penetrate the skin.[4]

Skin *absorption* occurs when a chemical enters through the top epidermis layer and remains somewhere between the middle and lower layers. Although bath-water can be absorbed through the top layer (causing a wrinkling effect), not all minerals found in water can penetrate the innermost hypodermis layer. Skin *penetration* occurs when a chemical breaks the skin barrier, breaches all three layers of the skin (epidermis, dermis and hypodermis) and reaches the bloodstream.

The health risks associated with chemicals penetrating the skin may be higher than consuming them in our diets, because when a toxic substance enters a man's digestive system, it's filtered through his kidneys and detoxified by his liver; but when toxins penetrate the skin, they bypass the liver's detoxification process and go directly into the bloodstream. That's why it's important to pay close attention to the ingredients listed on your personal hygiene products.

A good example of how toxic chemicals from personal hygiene products can cause serious health problems comes from the use of underarm deodorants and antiperspirants. Many antiperspirants contain an aluminum-based compound as the active ingredient, and they work when tiny fragments of aluminum pass through the skin's protective barrier and enter into the sweat pores, causing them to stop functioning properly. Not only do aluminum-based antiperspirants disable one of the body's detoxification methods, but aluminum is also a known carcinogen in animal studies and has been linked to Alzheimer's disease.

Some research suggests that aluminum-based compounds that penetrate the skin can cause estrogen-like hormonal effects. Because estrogen has the ability to promote the growth of breast cancer cells, some scientists believe that aluminum-based compounds in antiperspirants may contribute to the development of breast cancer. In an attempt to study this possibility more closely, researchers tested samples from breast-cancer patients who had undergone mastectomies. The women who used antiperspirants had deposits of aluminum in their outer breast tissue with higher concentrations of aluminum in the tissue closest to their underarms.[5]

Because aluminum is not normally found in the human body, it has prompted researchers to conduct more studies to determine if aluminum could interfere with a cell's ability to read its own DNA. While further research is being conducted, you may want to shop around for a more natural deodorant. Some options to consider would include a wide variety of organic personal care products found in most heath food stores.

Antibacterial Soap

Another common household product that may contain cancer-causing chemicals is soap. One man named Bill started buying a generic version of Softsoap® because it was cheap. Bill never read the label and he never had any concerns about the chemicals it contained or if those chemicals could be absorbed into his skin. Because Bill had purchased many containers of this clear hand soap, he filled all the soap dispensers in his house with it and even used it for shaving his face in the morning.

After many years of using what appeared to be a perfectly safe product, Bill began to notice red spots on his face that never seemed to heal. One possibility for the red spots was sun damage. In the past, Bill never took time to use sunscreen except for when he visited the beach. Another possibility could be some of the soap's antibacterial chemicals were being absorbed into his skin.

In an attempt to heal the red spots on his face, Bill tried natural remedies, including applying lime juice to the affected areas. He even purchased a natural skin repair product that contained aloe vera and green tea extract. Nothing seemed to help until he read the label on the bottle of his clear hand soap that clearly stated, "For External Use Only—Hands Only." Once Bill stopped using antibacterial soap on his face, the red spots began to heal.

In the event that your soap contains sodium laureth sulfate, diethanolamine, dioxane, triclosan, parabens, propylene glycol or synthetic colors, you may want to consider purchasing a more natural alternative. There are many options available at your local health food store, including fragrance-free glycerin soap for sensitive skin and liquid castile soap. More exotic varieties include sage lemongrass, sassafras birch, rosemary mint and black forest chamomile.

Another potentially toxic application for antibacterial soap is using it to wash fruits and vegetables. Antibacterial soaps may be effective for washing a cutting board after processing raw chicken meat, but when you wash tomatoes, grapes and leafy vegetables with it, the antibacterial chemicals can adhere to your produce, leaving behind a more toxic residue than what you are trying to wash off.

A better alternative for washing tomatoes, grapes or leafy vegetables would be to fill a spray bottle with vinegar. By applying one or two squirts to a tomato, the acid in the vinegar will start to dissolve the waxy pesticide residue, which can then be rinsed off with water a few minutes later. Other home remedies for cleaning produce include filling a spray bottle with one cup of water, one tablespoon of lemon juice and two tablespoons of baking soda.

To check the toxicity level of your personal care and cosmetic products, it's possible to conduct a search using the Environmental Working Group's database. By using the website's search function, you will be able to access more than 64,000 products using a chemical analysis system that will rate all the ingredients. Products that are rated below two are safe. Products rated between three and six pose a moderate hazard, and products rated above seven are high risk. For more information, please visit www.ewg.org.

Environmental Inspection

After evaluating the ingredients in your personal care and cosmetic products, you may want to conduct a careful examination of the other toxic chemicals inside your home. One man named George was using his basement to store automobile fluids, an old kerosene heater and some construction equipment. He had a rack in his storage room that contained many bottles of chemical solvents, antifreeze and motor oil.

Then one day, while George was working in the basement, he went to his storage room and found the bottle of lacquer thinner completely empty. He had purchased it over a year ago, and at that time, it was full. Even though the lid had been snapped on securely, the entire contents of the can had evaporated inside his house. The warning label read: "This product contains acetone, ethyl acetate, methanol, petroleum distillates and toluene. Cannot be made nonpoisonous. Using this product will expose you to chemicals which are known to the State of California to cause cancer and reproductive harm."

After George realized the entire can of lacquer thinner had evaporated inside his house, he cleaned out his storage room. Because George hadn't used the lacquer thinner in over a year, there wasn't any reason to store similar types of products inside his home, especially when the labels read "dangerous, flammable and extremely toxic." After thinking about his chemical exposure risk, George moved the kerosene heater into his garage, because even though it had a cover over the wick, kerosene could be drawn up through the wick and evaporate inside his house.

Other toxic cancer-causing fumes to avoid would include oven cleaner, cigarette smoke and diesel exhaust. The sign on gasoline pumps reads, "Long-term exposure to vapors has caused cancer in laboratory animals." In the event that you break an energy-saving, mercury lightbulb inside your house, the Environmental Protection Agency recommends vacating all people and animals from the room, shutting off the central heating and air-conditioning system, and ventilating the area to an outside air source for 10 minutes.[6]

After the area has been properly ventilated, the next step would be to clean up the broken glass. According to the EPA, you are not supposed to use a vacuum cleaner because it will only spread more toxic mercury particles in the air. The recommended way to clean up broken glass from a mercury lightbulb is to use sticky tape and damp paper towels. Afterward, the debris should be discarded in a sealed plastic bag and placed in an outdoor trash container.

Plastic Food Containers

After you have eliminated all the dangerous chemicals from your environment, the next step would be to evaluate your use of plastics. There are many different types of plastics, and each has been assigned a recycling code ranging between numbers one and seven. The manufacturers of recycling code three say that their products are *safer* than the manufacturers of recycling code number seven.

When there was a media alert several years ago about the dangers of BPA acting as a hormone disruptor, many of the manufacturers of recycling codes three, six and seven started making changes to the chemical compositions of their products. They began stamping "BPA-Free" on the plastic, even though the slightly altered chemical versions leach an even more harmful hormone disruptor.

Regardless of the manufacturer, the manufacturing process or the recycling code, all plastics are made from toxic chemicals. Because all plastics contain toxic chemicals, they will eventually break down over time, and when they break down, they will leach toxic chemicals into your environment. When plastic containers are used for culinary purposes, toxic chemicals can leach into your food and water, and when those chemicals are ingested, they can cause serious health problems.

For example, polycarbonate with recycling code seven is used to make food containers, baby bottles and water bottles. When heated and washed, polycarbonate plastic can break down and leach BPA. This toxic hormone disruptor has been linked to a number of health problems, including reproductive damage, early puberty and cancer.

Polyvinyl chloride with recycling code three is a softer pliable plastic. In order to make this plastic soft, phthalates are added during the manufacturing process. When phthalates leach out of the plastic, they can cause hormone disruption, reproductive disorders and liver cancer. According to the International Agency for Research on Cancer and the United States National Toxicology Program, phthalates are a known human carcinogen.[7]

Polystyrene with recycling code six is used to make meat trays, egg cartons, disposable cups and carryout containers. Polystyrene has been known to leach styrene, a neurotoxin and hormone disruptor. Styrene has been classified by the World Health Organization's International Agency for Research on Cancer as a possible human carcinogen.[8]

Although it will *not* be possible to eliminate plastics from your life, you can prevent the toxic chemicals from contaminating your food and water by using glass containers. There are many glass options available, including a 20-piece food storage set made by Pyrex that can also be used for baking. Another option would be using wide-mouth glass canning jars with airtight lids and half-gallon glass jars because they make excellent food storage containers.

While you are in the process of making your kitchen a safer, cancer-free environment, you may want to consider replacing all your plastic water bottles with stainless-steel containers. Another item you may want to replace would be any nonstick frying pans. Nonstick pans are coated with a synthetic polymer called *polytetrafluoroethylene,* and when it's overheated, the coating will emit toxic fumes. A better alternative would be to purchase stainless-steel or cast-iron cookware.

According to a study published by the *International Journal of Electrochemical Science,* the use of aluminum foil for food preparation is potentially toxic.[9] Aluminum foil may be safely used inside a refrigerator to create a makeshift lid on a large container, but when aluminum foil is heated, it will start to break apart. When aluminum foil is viewed under a microscope after it has been used to bake a potato, it's possible to see microscopic flakes of metal breaking away from the foil's surface. During the testing process, it didn't matter if the shiny or dull side of the foil was touching the potato, both sides contaminated the potato with a toxic amount of microscopic particles.

The Microwave Oven

Another dangerous kitchen cooking utensil you may want to stop using would be the microwave oven. It heats food by using electromagnetic energy. Inside every microwave oven there's a tube called a *magnetron,* where electrons are influenced by electromagnetic fields. Because microwaves use alternating current, they generate energy waves that alternate back and forth 60 times a second. When alternating energy waves interact with food, it causes molecular friction inside the food, and this friction is what heats up the food.

Applying molecular friction to food also creates toxic compounds because, when microwaves interact with the molecule structure of food, the friction deforms the molecules and tears them apart. The scientific term for this damage is called *structural isomerism*. In this process, naturally occurring amino acids have been observed undergoing isomeric changes. Microwaving food also creates new compounds called *radiolytic substances,* which are not found in nature.

To understand why creating radiolytic substances in food is harmful to your health, it may be helpful to compare the microwave cooking process to that of conventional heat. When a cup of water is boiled, thermal energy is added to the water molecules, causing them to speed up. In this process, *thermal* energy is converted into *kinetic* energy. When a person boils water, the water molecules speed up so fast they break apart (turn to steam) and evaporate into the air. The same laws of thermal dynamics also apply to convectional ovens.

When food is heated in an oven, thermal energy is transferred to the molecular structure causing different chemical reactions. For example, when heat is applied to egg whites, the molecular structure of the protein changes, and they become solid. When heat is applied to starches, they soften and swell. When heat is added to enzymes, it destroys their ability to perform chemical functions.

Thermal energy causes food molecules to expand as heat is applied from the outside, whereas electromagnetic energy shakes food molecules apart causing friction from within. Because both methods of cooking cause damage to the food's molecular structure, it may be helpful to discern which foods are more healthy eaten raw and which foods are more healthy when conventionally cooked.

Seeking God's Assistance

Because it is very easy to grow accustomed to the never-ending amount of toxins in our modern-day environment, it may be helpful to seek God's assistance to determine if there's anything that's causing problems to your health. A good example of being so close and familiar to a known carcinogen that most people would never suspect as the source of their medical problems comes from the birth control pill.

According to the International Agency for Research on Cancer, an arm of the World Health Organization, oral contraceptives, better known as *the pill*, have been classified as a group one carcinogen.[10] A group one classification has the highest risk rating and has been established as a known human carcinogen. Even though oral contraceptives have been proven to cause cancer, doctors continue to prescribe them to young girls for a variety of conditions, including acne, menstrual cramps, irregular menstrual cycles and birth control.

In the event that you have been suffering from a mysterious illness that no doctor can cure, you may want to spend some time in prayer seeking God's assistance. All you need to do is ask God to show you the source of your medical problems. For example, you may want to begin the process by praying, *Dear Heavenly Father, please show me if there's anything in my diet, personal care products, drinking water, medical prescriptions or environment that's causing harm to my health.*

After you ask God to show you the source, the next step would be to sit in silence and discern the answers. In the same way that Adam and Eve spent quiet time in nature, it may be helpful to visit a peaceful natural setting near a flowing stream. Another option would be to commune with God on a beach or in an open meadow surrounded by wildflowers.

As you discern the answers to your questions, you can rest assured that God loves you and has a purpose and plan for your life. God has already designed your body to naturally heal itself. By consuming a healthy diet of fresh organic fruits, vegetables, grains and seeds, you will be providing your body with all the healing nutrients that it needs.

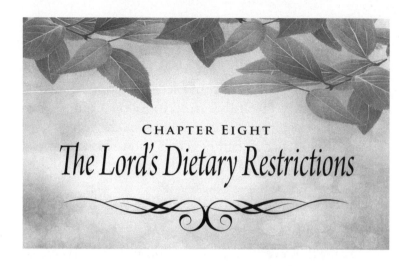

CHAPTER EIGHT

The Lord's Dietary Restrictions

After Adam had finished plowing the ground surrounding his home with the donkey's assistance, he planted the fields with millet, amaranth, black beans and buckwheat. A few months later, as summer was approaching, Eve conceived her first child. She gave birth to a beautiful boy whom she named Cain. The following spring, she gave birth to another precious child and named him Abel.

According to Genesis 4:2–5, *Abel was a keeper of sheep, and Cain a tiller of the ground. In the course of time Cain brought to the Lord an offering of the fruit of the ground, and Abel for his part brought of the firstlings of his flock, their fat portions. And the Lord had regard for Abel and his offering, but for Cain and his offering he had no regard. So Cain was very angry, and his countenance fell.*

Then the Lord said to Cain, *"Why are you angry, and why has your countenance fallen? If you do well, will you not be accepted? And if you do not do well, sin is lurking at the door; its desire is for you, but you must master it."*[1]

The very next day Cain said to his brother, *"Let us go out to the field."²* Abel could sense something was wrong, but he reluctantly agreed to follow Cain almost a mile past the almond orchard and into the forest. The seductive presence of darkness that had caused Adam and Eve's fall from grace was now pursuing Cain. The temptation was too strong. Soon after the brothers had entered a clearing, *Cain rose up against his brother Abel, and killed him.³*

Later that evening the Lord said to Cain, *"Where is your brother Abel?"⁴*

"I do not know; am I my brother's keeper?"⁵

The Lord said to him, *"What have you done? Listen; your brother's blood is crying out to me from the ground! And now you are cursed from the ground, which has opened its mouth to receive your brother's blood from your hand. When you till the ground, it will no longer yield to you its strength; you will be a fugitive and a wanderer on the earth."⁶*

Then Cain went away from the presence of the Lord, and settled in the land of Nod, east of Eden.⁷

Later that evening, God went over to Adam and Eve's house to tell them the bad news. After hearing how she lost both her boys in one day, Eve broke down and started to cry. During this time, God just held his beloved children as they sat in silence under a large oak tree.

Several chipmunks approached the grieving couple, followed by a family of gray rabbits and a herd of deer. The sad look in the eyes of Adam's donkey was apparent—he wanted to help, but because he didn't know what to do, he just drew close to Eve and offered his condolences in silence.

After a long time had passed, Eve wiped the tears from her eyes and said, "Why didn't you protect Abel?"

"I gave him many warnings," God said, "but he ignored them all."

"Then why didn't you stop Cain?" Adam asked.

"One of the greatest gifts that I have given humanity is their free will," God said. "Cain knew his actions were wrong, but it would also be wrong of me to violate his free will. If I followed Cain around all day with a whip to make sure he never did anything wrong, he wouldn't be free."

"Then how can we prevent these kind of tragedies from occurring in the future?" Eve asked.

"The best way would be to teach your descendants to respect my creation," God said.

"I can do that," Adam said. "I have been looking for additional work assignments. Maybe we could start by reaching out to Cain?"

"That's a good idea," God said. "Let's go to the land of Nod tomorrow to see how Cain is doing."

God's Law Concerning Blood

After the first murder had been committed, the seductive presence of darkness continued its deadly assault. In an attempt to prevent any more destruction from occurring, the Lord began issuing additional laws by saying, *"For your own lifeblood I will surely require a reckoning: from every animal I will require it and from human beings, each one for the blood of another, I will require a reckoning for human life."*[8]

"For the life of the flesh is in the blood; and I have given it to you for making atonement for your lives on the altar; for, as life, it is the blood that makes atonement. It shall be a perpetual statute throughout your generations, in all your settlements: you must not eat any fat or any blood."[9]

After God issued laws concerning the shedding and consumption of blood, the seductive presence of darkness began inciting humanity to consume as much blood as possible. For example, one popular blood sausage recipe is made from boiled pig's blood and mixed with pieces of pork fat. After spices are added, the mixture is stuffed into sausage casings and served grilled or sautéed with garlic.

There are also many people living in Africa today that will drink blood directly from a cow. In the Maasai tribe, several men will hold a cow's head while another man fastens a tourniquet around the animal's neck. When a large vein appears, one of the men will stab the vein with a knife, creating a small puncture. Because of the built-up pressure, blood will start flowing out faster than a drinking fountain. After a one-liter bottle has been filled, the men will slide the tourniquet over the wound to stop the bleeding.

From the Maasai's perspective, there's nothing wrong with drinking blood from a cow. After giving two quarts of blood once a month, the cow recovers and is able to make another donation in the future. Because the Maasai spend a lot of time and effort providing pasture for their cows to graze, they consider it the cow's obligation to either produce milk or blood for them to consume.

After God gave strict laws concerning the consumption of blood, he also gave humanity a list of animals that should never be eaten. For example, in the book of Leviticus 11:27, God said, *"All that walk on their paws, among the animals that walk on all fours, are unclean for you."* This would include the consumption of cats, dogs, hyenas, leopards, gorillas, chimpanzees or any other type of monkey. God gave humanity these dietary restrictions because there are many dangerous pathogens and viruses that live inside of animals.

One strain of virus that can live its entire lifetime inside a monkey has been named the *human immunodeficiency virus.* When HIV jumped species due to a violation of God's laws through the consumption of bush meat, a wave of destruction was released. The destruction began the day a hunter captured a monkey and decided to eat its flesh. As the man was butchering the animal, some of the monkey's blood entered the tiny cuts on the man's hands and allowed the virus to jump species. After the man contracted AIDS, he spread the disease to different sexual partners, and now there are millions of AIDS orphans living in Africa.

The same situation has also occurred with the Ebola virus. According to Leviticus 11:13–19, God said, *"These you shall regard as detestable among the birds. They shall not be eaten; they are an abomination: the eagle, the vulture, the osprey, the buzzard, the kite of any kind; every raven of any kind; the ostrich, the nighthawk, the sea gull, the hawk of any kind; the little owl, the cormorant, the great owl, the water hen, the desert owl, the carrion vulture, the stork, the heron of any kind, the hoopoe, and the bat."*

After the first Ebola outbreak occurred in 1976, scientists were able to trace the disease back to a man who purchased a fruit bat from the local market. After taking the bat home, he butchered the animal and ate the meat for dinner. A few days later, he contracting the Ebola virus and spread the disease to his daughter. The Ebola virus can live its entire lifetime inside a bat without causing harm, but when viruses jump species, disastrous consequences can be expected.

According to the United States Department of Defense, the cost to stop the 2014 Ebola outbreak has already exceeded $330 million.[10] The majority of the money the United States spent was used to build a temporary hospital in Monrovia, along with 10 other treatment centers throughout Liberia. The United States military also trained over 1,500 health care workers, provided thousands of hazmat suits and set up mobile testing laboratories. If it wasn't for the intervention of many countries, including Australia, Germany, Sweden, Japan and China, the Ebola virus could have swept across the entire continent of Africa, killing the majority of its inhabitants, all because of one man's desire to eat bush meat.

God's Law Concerning Pork

Other forbidden foods include winged insects, bugs, mice, rats, rabbits, lizards, frogs, crocodiles and the pig. According to Leviticus 11:7–8, God said, *"The pig, for even though it has divided hoofs and is cleft-footed, it does not chew the cud; it is unclean for you. Of their flesh you shall not eat, and their carcasses you shall not touch; they are unclean for you."*

The main reason why God declared pigs unclean is that they go around all day eating garbage. In Africa, pigs are herded from their owner's homes in the morning to the local trash dump where they dig through garbage looking for food. It's also possible to watch pigs wallowing around in open sewers, looking for human waste to consume.

Although the practice of feeding garbage to hogs has been outlawed in the United States since 1980, it's still possible to apply for a garbage-feeding permit. According to the United States Department of Agriculture, there are over 2,700 licensed and regulated garbage-feeding pig farms in operation today in 29 states.[11] The farmers are required to heat the waste products to 212 degrees for 30 minutes before feeding the slop to the animals.

The cooking process is designed to kill viruses in the garbage that could make the pigs sick. Because hogs are particularly susceptible to disease, it's important to keep them healthy, because if one pig gets sick, the animal could spread the disease to other livestock. Once a pig becomes infected with foot-and-mouth disease, African swine fever or trichinosis, the viruses and pathogens can remain dormant inside the pig's flesh even after the meat has been chilled, frozen or cured.

Although the garbage-cooking process is designed to kill viruses that could make pigs sick, it doesn't eliminate any toxic chemicals from the pig's diets. A good example of toxic chemicals that are fed to pigs comes from a farmer who purchases industrial waste from an ice cream manufacturing facility. The chemical slop that he feeds the animals looks similar to the sticky remains of imitation ice cream that has been left out under the hot sun all day.

When fed garbage its entire lifetime, the pig's body will use those chemicals to build every cell in its body. Not only have most of the chemicals, preservatives and food colorings that are used to make imitation ice cream been proven to cause cancer in laboratory animals, they can also cause cancer in pigs.

When a pig eats an unhealthy diet of toxic waste its entire lifetime, toxins can build up in the pig's fat cells, causing some of those cells to mutate. When this occurs, rebellious cells can take on a life of their own. Refusing to die, they will start fermenting sugars to live longer.

Once the mutated cells spread throughout the pig's body, a highly aggressive form of cancer can develop. If the pig starts looking unhealthy, the farmer will usually rush the animal off to market before it dies. After a meat processing plant purchases the commodity, it will be infused with nitrates and other cancer-causing chemicals. The end result is then sold in grocery stores across the nation.

Pork Contains Parasitic Worms

Another reason God doesn't want his beloved children eating pork is to prevent parasitic worms from destroying a person's health. A good example of the dangers of eating pork comes from a young woman named Sarah who thought she had a brain tumor. Her symptoms started with a small amount of numbness in her left arm. When Sarah started experiencing balancing problems and difficulty swallowing, she knew something was seriously wrong, so she immediately checked herself into the emergency room.

The MRI scan revealed a foreign growth in her brain that looked like a tumor, so the doctors scheduled an operation. During the operation, the surgeon discovered a parasitic worm that had been eating her brain. After the surgeon removed it, Sarah woke up from the operating table to hear the good news—she didn't have a tumor after all, only a pork tapeworm called *taenia solium*.

If you are wondering how a tapeworm could pass through Sarah's stomach and enter her brain, the journey begins with a parasite called *cysticercosis* that lives in pork. When a person eats undercooked pork, it's possible to consume some of the parasite's larva. These tiny worms are very small and can survive extreme temperatures for an extended period of time. Once the baby worms pass through a person's digestive system, they will enter the large intestine, where they will attach themselves to the inner walls and start feeding.

After the baby worms grow into an adult tapeworm, they can produce up to 50,000 eggs. Most of these eggs pass directly through a person's colon and end up in the toilet, but in the event the host doesn't wash his or her hands properly, it's possible to accidentally consume some of the tapeworm's eggs. In the event that a person accidentally consumes just one tiny egg, the egg is so small that it can pass directly through a person's stomach and enter his or her bloodstream.

Once inside the bloodstream, the egg can travel anywhere in that person's body, including the brain. Once the eggs hatch, tiny worms will start feeding on the host's flesh. In an attempt to prevent his beloved children from experiencing the destructive consequences of parasitic worms, God has given his beloved children a very simple rule concerning pork by saying, *"their flesh you shall not eat, and their carcasses you shall not touch; they are unclean for you."* [12]

Interpretation of God's Law

Because God has made it clear that he doesn't want his beloved children eating pork or touching pigs without washing their hands, you may be wondering how Jesus could declare all foods clean. The verse is stated in Mark 7:18–20, when Jesus said, *"Do you not see that whatever goes into a person from outside cannot defile, since it enters, not the heart but the stomach, and goes out into the sewer?" (Thus he declared all foods clean.) And he said, "It is what comes out of a person that defiles."*

To study the meaning of this passage, it may be helpful to start at the beginning of the chapter when the Pharisees accused the Lord's disciples of eating with defiled hands. According to Mark 7:1–2, *When the Pharisees and some of the scribes who had come from*

Jerusalem gathered around him, they noticed that some of his disciples were eating with defiled hands, that is, without washing them. So the Pharisees and the scribes asked him, "Why do your disciples not live according to the tradition of the elders, but eat with defiled hands?" [13]

In an attempt to focus the religious leader's attention on the meaning of spiritual defilement, Jesus said, *"For it is from within, from the human heart, that evil intentions come: fornication, theft, murder, adultery, avarice, wickedness, deceit, licentiousness, envy, slander, pride, folly. All these evil things come from within, and they defile a person."* [14]

The Lord's entire conversation with the Pharisees was focused on what spiritually defiles a person before God. The Hebrew word for *defile* (גָּאַל) and the Greek word for *defile* (κοινόω) both mean to make unholy, polluted or profane. To further clarify this point, Jesus *called the crowd again and said to them, "Listen to me, all of you, and understand: there is nothing outside a person that by going in can defile, but the things that come out are what defile."* [15]

When he had left the crowd and entered the house, his disciples asked him about the parable. He said to them, "Then do you also fail to understand? Do you not see that whatever goes into a person from outside cannot defile, since it enters, not the heart but the stomach, and goes out into the sewer?" [16]

After studying the Lord's conversation with the Pharisees, it's easy to see that the correct interpretation is that spiritual defilement does not occur by eating kosher or nonkosher foods, but rather, spiritual defilement occurs through our sinful actions. In the same way that it's not possible to enter into an authentic relationship with God by following a list of kosher dietary restrictions, it's also not possible to spiritually defile yourself before God just because you ate a rabbit for dinner.

God has given us his dietary restrictions because he loves us and wants to protect us from sickness and disease. When a man eats beef that has been infected with mad cow disease, he will get sick because the normal cooking process does not kill the prions that contaminate the cow's flesh. When a man eats tapeworm eggs, the tiny organisms can pass through his stomach, circulate throughout his body and end up eating parts of his brain.

Combining Milk & Meat Together

Another dietary restriction that has been issued in Exodus 23:19 says, *You shall not boil a kid in its mother's milk.* If you were to ask a Jewish rabbi to explain the meaning of this passage, he would probably say the commandment has significant importance to God because it has been listed in Scripture three different times: Exodus 23:19, Exodus 34:26 and Deuteronomy 14:21.

The rabbi may go on to explain that because God's children have been instructed *not* to cook with milk and meat together, then God doesn't want his children consuming milk and meat together during the same meal. And furthermore, if God doesn't want his beloved children cooking with milk and meat, then we should not try to indulge our sensual pleasures (debauchery) by consuming milk and meat during the same meal.

For example, if a rabbi drinks a glass of milk for breakfast, he must wait one hour before consuming meat. If the rabbi consumes meat for lunch, he must wait six hours before consuming dairy products. The same law of separation also applies to pots and pans. If a man cooks chicken in a new saucepan, the pan becomes designated for meat. If the man were to heat milk in the same saucepan, the *fleishik* properties of the pan would transfer to the *milchik* contents of the liquid, and both the milk and the pan would be considered unclean for future use.

Although most people would consider the separation of pots and pans a little extreme, there are plenty of good reasons why God does not want his beloved children combining certain foods together during the same meal. For example, when a man drinks a glass of milk, his stomach produces a digestive enzyme called *rennin* that causes the coagulation of milk. Rennin also releases minerals from the milk and changes the milk into a usable form of protein.

When a man consumes meat and potatoes, his gallbladder releases bile and his stomach produces hydrochloric acid to break down the meat, while his pancreas releases amylases that split apart starches and lipases to split apart fats. A man's pancreas will also produce ribonuclease, deoxyribonuclease and gelatinase to ensure that everything is assimilated properly.

When a man consumes dairy and meat together during the same meal, his digestive system needs to process two different forms of protein at the same time. Because dairy products require the coagulation of milk and meat requires proteases to break down the proteins, the human digestive system will function more smoothly when a person consumes only one form of protein at a time.

Other food combinations that are difficult to digest would be grapefruit juice and milk. The acid-based juice will cause an adverse reaction with the milk. The same would be true if you tried eating baking soda and vinegar. An adverse chemical reaction between the acid and alkaline compounds would occur.

Combining Protein & Starches Together

A good example of how mixing certain foods together during the same meal can cause digestive problems comes from a man named Jack who used to consume an all-American diet. When Jack was in his late twenties, his diet consisted mostly of macaroni and cheese, hot dogs, spaghetti and meatballs, hamburgers and pizza. During this time, Jack would experience painful stomach cramps and heartburn.

In an attempt to treat his acid reflux, Jack would try different antacid medications, but nothing seemed to help. Then one day, while Jack was visiting his friend's house, he noticed a small food-combining chart posted on his friend's refrigerator. He was curious about the chart's meaning, so after making an inquiry, his friend said, "It will wipe out indigestion. When you stop combining proteins and starches, you will never have heartburn again."

Jack was so excited that he borrowed his friend's chart and started applying the principles to his life. Within the first 24 hours, Jack started to feel better.

He continued following the chart's instructions for a full week and couldn't believe the results. His stomach cramps and painful burning sensation in the back of his throat had completely disappeared.

Because Jack couldn't believe the results, he decided to go back to his all-American diet of mixing different forms of protein and starches together during the same meal. As soon as he reverted back to his old eating habits, his painful stomach cramps returned. As Jack pondered the results, he realized that he didn't have any control over the amount of hydrochloric acid that his stomach produced, or any control over the digestive enzymes his pancreas released, but he *did* have control over what kind of foods he placed inside his body.

Jack also started pondering the wisdom of taking antacid drugs to solve a digestive problem. For example, if every time a man consumed baking soda and vinegar he experienced stomach cramps, the logical conclusion would be to stop mixing those chemicals together. Since science would support the fact that the problem was being caused by an acid and alkaline reaction, to solve the problem, the answer would consist of less toxic food combinations, not more antacid drugs and chemicals.

After Jack concluded his experiment with the all-American diet, he went back and applied the rules of the food-combining chart to his life for another week, only this time he applied them with an increased amount of thoughtfulness and seriousness. Once again, the results were astounding, and Jack was sold. After he stopped combining proteins and starches together in the same meal, his digestive problems were forever resolved.

It took Jack about a year to make all the final adjustments to his diet, but he eventually settled on eating fruits in the morning, followed by vegetables and starches in the afternoon, and vegetables and proteins for dinner. Other options would include eating fruits in the morning, followed by vegetables and grains, followed by vegetables and meats. In Jack's situation, he also found it helpful to consume all fruits separately.

Because every person's digestive system will function and react differently, you may want to spend some time in prayer asking God if there are any food combinations that are causing problems to your health. It's a very simple prayer: *Dear Heavenly Father, please show me if I'm consuming any adverse food combinations that are causing problems to my health.*

It would also be possible to ask the Lord a few simple questions and then sit in silence and meditate on his answers. A good prayer to start with would be, *Dear Heavenly Father, do you want me to stop mixing meat and dairy products together during the same meal?* Another question to ask would be, *Do you want me to separate meats from starches?*

Avoiding Foods with Fungus

Another consideration for a healthy diet would be to avoid foods that are susceptible to mold and fungus. This would include peanuts, because they grow underground and have been known to contain over 20 different strains of fungus.

Another example of food that has been contaminated with fungus comes from barley. Although barley is an ancient grain, it is also highly susceptible to fungus. One way to put barley to the test is to soak some in hydrogen peroxide. You will quickly discover that a teaspoon of barley mixed with hydrogen peroxide will foam for more than 10 minutes.

When you test other whole grains such as millet, amaranth and quinoa, you may notice a small amount of bacterial cleansing, but it will not react like barley. That's because other grains have harder exterior shells that make them more resistant to bacterial and fungal infections. Because barley has weaker natural defenses, fungus can enter into the grain and produce mycotoxins that can cause health problems in both animals and humans.

Another example of a popular product that you may want to avoid is blue cheese, because it has been injected with mold to give it a distinct flavor. Although you can kill many types of mold by heating them at 212 degrees for 30 minutes, the toxins and waste products the mold produces will not disappear once the mold is dead.

Another experiment that you can conduct with hydrogen peroxide involves mushrooms. In the event that you have mushrooms growing in your backyard, you may have noticed a semi-circular root system, often called a *fairy ring*. When the underground root system produces a seed-dispersing fruit, it sprouts up in the form of mushrooms. If you have mushrooms growing in your backyard, you can cut one into pieces and soak it in hydrogen peroxide. You may also want to cut up a store-bought mushroom and soak it in hydrogen peroxide to see which one contains more mycotoxins.

God's Law Concerning Seafood

Another important dietary restriction concerning seafood comes from Leviticus 11:9–11, when God said, *"Everything in the waters that has fins and scales, whether in the seas or in the streams—such you may eat. But anything in the seas or the streams that does not have fins and scales, of the swarming creatures in the waters and among all the other living creatures that are in the waters—they are detestable to you and detestable they shall remain."*

Forbidden forms of seafood include bottom-feeding scavengers like crawfish, catfish, clams, crabs, lobster, shrimp, mussels, oysters, scallops, squid, snails and frogs. Although catfish have fins, they do not have scales, and therefore are a forbidden source of food. Although lobsters and crabs may be considered a delicacy for many people, they are bottom-feeding scavengers and a member of the arthropod family that also includes cockroaches, caterpillars and spiders.

If you have ever noticed the tiny black line running down the backside of shrimp—it's part of the shrimp's colon. The actual colon is a clear tube. The black content inside the clear tube is the shrimp's feces. On a rare occasion, you may find a shrimp with an empty colon, but the majority of the time, the colon is stuffed with all the garbage they have been eating. After all, shrimp are ocean floor garbage collectors. The contents of a shrimp's colons have been known to contain parts of insects, rat hairs and chemical residue from commercial farming operations.

Acceptable forms of seafood would include bluefish, butterfish, cod, flounder, haddock, halibut, herring, mackerel, pike, red snapper, salmon, sardine, sea bass, smelt, sole, trout and whitefish. Although tuna has fins and scales, you may want to remove it from your diet due to its high mercury content. According to warnings issued by the United States Food and Drug Administration and the Environmental Protection Agency, the high mercury content found in shark, swordfish, king mackerel and tuna can harm a young child's nervous system.[17]

The majority of the mercury in our oceans comes from air pollution that's emitted by coal-fired power plants. After the heavy metal rises into our atmosphere, it settles upon the ocean's surface in the form of methyl-mercury, where it contaminates all forms of marine life. When larger fish eat smaller fish, they accumulate higher levels of mercury in their bodies. Because tuna, shark, swordfish and king mackerel eat a lot of smaller fish and have longer life spans, they acquire more mercury in their bodies.

There are two main types of tuna sold in grocery stores today, *chunk light* and *albacore*. Most albacore tuna has three times the amount of mercury than the smaller skipjack species that is used in chunk light. Albacore tuna contains 0.32 parts per million of mercury, whereas chunk light contains 0.12 parts per million of mercury. A better alternative to tuna would be canned salmon. The best choice would be wild sockeye or wild pink salmon from Alaska.

Farm-Raised Fish

Another consideration for a safe and healthy diet would be to avoid farm-raised fish. According to studies conducted by the Environmental Working Group, the cancer-causing chemical known as *polychlorinated Biphenyl* was 16 times higher in farm-raised salmon compared to those caught in the wild.[18] Researchers have also found higher levels of *polybrominated diphenyl ether,* a chemical used as a flame retardant, in farm-raised fish. Another study conducted by the University of New York found dioxin levels in farm-raised salmon to be 11 times higher compared to those caught wild.[19] Dioxins have the ability to impair a person's immune, nervous and reproductive systems and are known carcinogens.

Another reason to avoid farm-raised salmon can be found printed on the packaging in tiny letters that state, "color added." If you are wondering how it's possible to add coloring to salmon, there's a synthetic pigment called *canthaxanthin* that is added to the fish's diet. Wild salmon develop their deep red color through a natural diet of eating krill, but farm-raised salmon are so sick and unhealthy from eating garbage all day that their flesh is a dirty gray color. Because consumers would never purchase dirty gray salmon, the same chemical compound that's used in sunless tanning pills is being added to the fish's food supply.

Farm-raised fish are also fed growth hormones and treated with antibiotics to prevent disease. They are also treated with pesticides that are used to kill sea lice. Maybe the most disturbing reason why you should avoid eating farm-raised fish is that they are fed chicken and pig feces. According to the director of the University of Georgia's Center for Food Safety, "The manure the Chinese use to feed fish is frequently contaminated with microbes like salmonella."[20]

When confronted with this concern, the chairman of a government-sponsored Tilapia Aquaculture Association in Lianjiang, China, said that he "discourages using feces as food because it contaminates water and makes fish more susceptible to diseases." But because of fierce competition, "a growing number of Guangdong farmers adopt that practice anyways."[21] Many farmers have switched to feces and have stopped using commercial feed altogether.

By purifying your drinking water, eliminating toxic chemicals from your environment and following the Lord's dietary restrictions, you will be empowering and strengthening your immune system. By giving your body plenty of rest, reducing stress and spending time developing a deeper relationship with the Lord, you will be better prepared to overcome any kind of illness through the unlimited power of God himself.

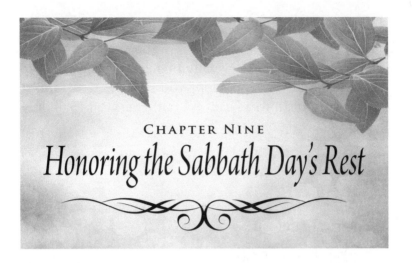

CHAPTER NINE

Honoring the Sabbath Day's Rest

It was a bright and beautiful morning in the garden when Adam and Eve found themselves worried about Belle, a black-and-white heifer that was about to give birth. The other animals knew Belle was in a great deal of agony. Her yawning moans could be heard throughout the night. A herd of deer had drawn close to keep her company, while several gray rabbits darted back and forth.

Adam and Eve had never experienced anything like this before. Belle had entered a patch of scrub oak near the stream. She was surrounded by tall grass, lying on her side trying to give birth, but the calf's life was in danger.

Eve instinctually rushed to the mother's side and very gently started pulling on the calf's hind legs. It took about 15 minutes, but after the calf had been set free, Belle rose to her feet and began licking her newborn baby.

Later that evening, Adam and Eve couldn't wait to see God. When they heard him walking in the garden during the time of the evening breeze, they rushed to meet him. "We're so happy you're here," Eve said. "Belle gave birth to a beautiful calf. Everything's fine, but we needed your help."

"I was with you," God said, "watching over every detail."

"But we were so worried something bad would happen," Adam said.

"Yes, I know," God said. "I designed you to respond that way. Do you remember our conversation when the forest caught fire?"

"Yes," Adam said as he looked down.

"Don't worry," God said. "You both did an excellent job!"

Although life in the garden was mostly peaceful, there were many occasions when Adam and Eve needed to respond to stressful situations. One of the worst events occurred when lightning struck and set the forest ablaze.

When Adam first sensed danger, his nervous system released a flood of hormones, including adrenaline and cortisol. Within a split second, his heartbeat increased, muscles tightened, blood pressure rose, and his senses became sharper and more clearly focused.

All these internal changes occurred to increase Adam's physical strength, speed, stamina and reaction time, preparing him to either fight the dangerous fire or give him the necessary strength to run away.

The Fight-or-Flight Response

Although God designed Adam and Eve's bodies perfectly, the human nervous system cannot distinguish between real threats and imaginary circumstances. If Adam simply imagined the forest had been set ablaze, or if he sat around worrying what would happen if the forest had caught fire, adrenaline and cortisol would be released into his bloodstream, creating the same fight-or-flight response.

If this were to occur, Adam's digestive system would shut down so that more blood could be delivered to his muscles. If the threat were only imaginary, Adam's body would be revved up for high performance, but because no action was necessary, his body would need to rebalance those hormones and restart his digestive system later that evening.

As you can imagine, Adam could cause a lot of damage to his body by constantly thinking stressful thoughts when no actions were necessary. If Adam sat around all day worrying about everything that could go wrong with God's creation, he may soon develop digestive problems. An excessive amount of cortisol in his bloodstream would cause his body to store unnecessary fat. If Adam tried to comfort his stressful emotions by overeating when his digestive system had shut down, he may experience indigestion and stomach cramps.

Because of an elevated heart rate during the fight-or-flight response, Adam would also be more likely to experience strokes and heart attacks. The excessive amount of adrenaline and other hormones in Adam's body would raise his blood sugar levels, causing migraine headaches and even interfering with his ability to experience a peaceful night's sleep. Other destructive consequences would include premature aging, hair loss and a weakened immune system.

To further understand the harmful effects of stress on the human body, it may be helpful to compare it to an automobile. For example, picture what it would be like driving on a winding mountain road through a densely populated pine tree forest. Although it's a hot and dry summer's day, the soft mountain breeze has gradually turned into a strong windstorm. As the sky grows dark, lightning strikes, and before long the entire forest is set ablaze. There's only one road leading to safety, but thick, billowing smoke makes it impossible to see where you're going.

Scorching flames towering hundreds of feet high consume large trees, causing them to fall across the road and block your escape route. In this situation, it would be appropriate to allow your thoughts to perceive the worst possible scenario. The looming threat is very dangerous and extremely serious. The proper response would be to start your car's engine, punch the accelerator to the floor and get out of there as fast as possible.

Now picture the same car parked safely in your garage. There's no fire. There's no real threat or danger, but you still have the gas peddle pressed to the floor. The car is not moving but the motor is shaking itself apart, spinning at over 7,000 RPM. Day after day, your car's engine is producing an extreme amount of heat and vibration, but there's no real workload being applied to the motor or transmission.

In the same way that the motor of a brand-new car would destroy itself after being treated in this manner, so too will the human body when exposed to stress hormones on a regular basis. When a man thinks stressful thoughts, his nervous system responds by releasing hormones that allow his body to run at an extremely high output level. This function works great when there's an actual emergency that requires action, but when no action is required, stress has the ability to destroy a person's health in a very short amount of time.

In an effort to prevent the destructive consequences of stress from harming Adam and Eve's bodies, God would commune with his beloved children on a regular basis. God wanted Adam and Eve to know when it was appropriate to depress the accelerator to the floor and when to turn off the ignition. This process begins by evaluating your thoughts on a regular basis, and when necessary, to stop thinking about the worst possible scenario and convert those thoughts into praise, worship and thanksgiving.

Taking Every Thought Captive

A good example on how to take every thought captive comes from the book of Philippians, which says, *Rejoice in the Lord always; again I will say, Rejoice. Let your gentleness be known to everyone. The Lord is near. Do not worry about anything, but in everything by prayer and supplication with thanksgiving let your requests be made known to God. Finally, beloved, whatever is true, whatever is honorable, whatever is just, whatever is pure, whatever is pleasing, whatever is commendable, if there is any excellence and if there is anything worthy of praise, think about these things.*[1]

To put this Scripture passage into practice, it may be helpful to identify three areas of stress in your life. What are the three greatest concerns that you are constantly worrying about? _____ _____ & _____

The next step would be to offer praise and worship to God for any positive aspects of these situations. How have these situations helped you learn, grow and make changes in life? What are the positive aspects that you can be thankful for? _____ _____ & _____

The next step would be to spend time in prayer and ask God to show you what actions he wants you to take. How would the Lord want you to respond? _____ & _____ _____ & _____

Because there were many times in Adam and Eve's lives when they found it extremely difficult to take every thought captive, God also required a full and complete day of rest. The Sabbath day allowed God's children the necessary time to commune with their Creator and ask questions regarding the stressful circumstances that they were facing.

In addition to providing wisdom and knowledge during this time, the Sabbath also served as a safeguard to protect their health. In the event that God's children became so consumed with their daily affairs (constantly revving their motors), the Sabbath day would require the physical removal of the keys from the car's ignition.

That way, when they were going through a stressful season in life, they would not destroy their health with excessive engine heat. The Sabbath would also provide them with 52 mini-vacations per year.

The concept for a full and complete day of rest was originally established by God when he created the heavens and earth. According to Genesis 2:2–3, *On the seventh day God finished the work that he had done, and he rested on the seventh day from all the work that he had done. So God blessed the seventh day and hallowed it, because on it God rested from all the work that he had done in creation.*

God also issued a command to all of Adam and Eve's descendants in the book of Exodus, as follows: *Remember the Sabbath day, and keep it holy. Six days you shall labor and do all your work. But the seventh day is a Sabbath to the Lord your God; you shall not do any work— you, your son or your daughter, your male or female slave, your livestock, or the alien resident in your towns. For in six days the Lord made heaven and earth, the sea, and all that is in them, but rested the seventh day; therefore the Lord blessed the Sabbath day and consecrated it.* [2]

Honoring God's Commandments

Because the Lord rested on the seventh day, the Sabbath has been traditionally observed beginning Friday evening and continuing until Saturday evening. If you were to ask a Jewish rabbi at what hour the Sabbath begins, he might say, "When you can hold up two strings toward the evening twilight—one white and one black—as soon as you cannot tell the difference in color, it's the Sabbath." Another way to know when the Sabbath begins is by observing three stars in the evening sky. When it's dark enough to see several stars in the evening twilight, it's time to stop working and begin a sacred time of rest.

Although the Sabbath has been traditionally honored on the seventh day of the week for many centuries, because Jesus rose from the dead on the first day of the week, many first-century Christians began celebrating the *Lord's Day* on Sunday. As the division widened between the first-century Christians and the Jews, many people slowly gave up their observance of the seventh day and began meeting for worship on the first day of the week.

Although instructions for the Sabbath day's rest may be easy to understand, they are usually very difficult to follow. It an attempt to make it easier, Jewish rabbis have designed an elaborate system of laws. For example, if you were to visit Israel on the Sabbath, you may find the elevators stopping on every floor when no one has pressed the buttons. The elevators have been programmed this way so that people can ride them without doing any work.

Although many people would consider the rule of no-button-pushing on the Sabbath a little extreme, it would appear by our fast-paced, stressed-out society that some rules for rest are not only important, but also necessary. The main purpose for the Sabbath is to spend a full day of rest communing with God. This means that you should finish all your work assignments, chores and activities the day before. The Sabbath is a special time to be with God, almost like a date between lovers that look forward to spending time together.

For many people the Sabbath is best spent praying, meditating, walking in nature, studying Scripture and sleeping. Although it's extremely difficult for some people to rest all day without engaging in some kind of activity (like washing clothes and checking email), spending a full day with God is the best possible use of our time here on earth. After spending a full day of rest in God's presence, you will be spiritually refreshed, filled with wisdom and insight, and raring to get back to work the following morning.

A good example of how it's possible to honor the Sabbath without ever being able to commune with God comes from a man named Carlos who made plans to visit the beach. During this time, Carlos had been fasting all week on juice and water in a small town in Mexico. Because the Sabbath was approaching, Carlos thought it would be nice to spend the day at the beach communing with the Lord. After attending church on Sunday, Carlos parked his vehicle and boarded a bus.

Carlos didn't want to drive his personal vehicle to the beach because it was located on a secluded part of the coast and the roads leading to the beach were extremely rough. About an hour into the journey, Carlos started to regret his decision. Not only was the bus crowded and slow, but there was a large hole near the engine compartment that allowed smoke and exhaust fumes to enter the vehicle. A journey that would have taken an hour in his personal vehicle turned out to be twice as long.

After a long and painful bus ride, Carlos was hoping to find a beautiful white sandy beach where he could spend the day communing with the Lord. Instead, Carlos discovered a rocky shoreline littered with trash and seaweed. To make matters worse, storm clouds had covered the sun and it started to rain. Because Carlos was cold and didn't feel like swimming, he wrapped himself in a towel and took shelter on the side of a dilapidated wooden shack.

Because the public bus only serviced that remote location twice a day, Carlos had to wait a very long time for the next bus to arrive. He spent most of the day on the side of the wooden shack. When Carlos finally returned home, he was exhausted. His spiritual day at the beach turned out to be a disaster. The fast made his body weak, and although he had good intentions, he wasn't able to spend very much quality time communing with the Lord. The experience taught Carlos a very valuable lesson—the Sabbath day needs to be a time of rest and refreshment with the Lord.

The very next weekend, Carlos decided to spend the entire Sabbath resting with the Lord. After attending church on Sunday, he spent the rest of the day enjoying the simplicity of silence. He didn't go shopping, check email, watch television, do laundry or attend any sporting events; instead, he spent time mediating on the Lord's will for his life, reading his Bible, praying and sleeping. When Monday morning arrived, he was fully rested, refreshed and ready to get back to work.

God gave us the Sabbath as a full and complete day of rest. It's a time to commune with the Lord, ask questions about the direction of our lives and spend the necessary time in silence discerning God's answers. It's also a time for our bodies to rest, recover, rebalance and be restored to good health.

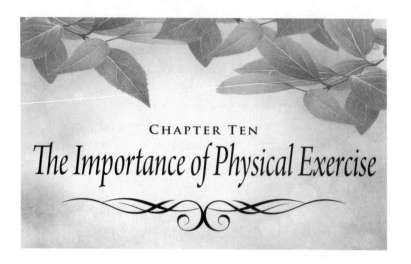

CHAPTER TEN

The Importance of Physical Exercise

When God created the universe, he simply spoke it into existence. In order to understand how that was possible, it may be helpful to picture an atom. If you magnified an atom to the size of a football field, the nucleus would be the size of a marble, and there would be a series of electrons and protons spinning around the nucleus in perfect harmony. As you gaze upon this incredible phenomena, you may find yourself wondering—how is that possible? Where do electrons get the energy to make a perpetual orbital rotation around the nucleus?

In an attempt to discover the answer, scientists have built the Large Hadron Collider located on the borders of France and Switzerland. It's the largest machine in the world and has the ability to send proton beams traveling in opposite directions around a 17-mile tunnel buried hundreds of feet underground. The protons travel a little slower than the speed of light and can make 11,000 revolutions around the tunnel per second.

There are seven detectors located in underground caverns that study the results of the particle collisions.

One detector called *ATLAS* is looking for the origins of mass and extra dimensions. Another detector called *CMS* is looking for the Higgs boson, or the God particle. Many of these scientists want to understand the Big Bang theory better. Others want to know what gives molecules their mass, while others want to discover dark matter or the invisible source that brings all things to life.

According to Colossians 1:16–17, *All things in heaven and on earth were created, things visible and invisible, whether thrones or dominions or rulers or powers—all things have been created through him and for him. He himself is before all things, and in him all things hold together.*

When God created Adam and Eve's bodies, he breathed the *breath of life* into their molecular structure and they became living beings.[1] Because every cell in the human body is comprised of atoms, it may be helpful to understand how atoms form molecular machines. After we explore how molecular machines function, it will be easier to understand why physical exercise is important to our health.

Molecular Machines

To begin with, there are trillions of cells inside the human body. At this very moment, your brain cells are allowing you to read the words on this page. Your liver cells are purging toxic chemicals from your body, while other cells are making fuel and fighting off bacteria. The molecular machines inside the human body all function together in perfect harmony while accomplishing different assignments. Some of our cells operate as chemical factories, while others form a transportation grid and communications network.

Every cell in the human body contains a nucleus, which serves as the cell's brain. The nucleus contains the cell's genetic code, which determines the cell's identity and predetermines all its activities. Cells also need to generate their own power source. Most cells use a rechargeable process called *adenosine triphosphate* or *ATP*.

This process creates energy when a rechargeable molecular unit called *adenosine* is coupled together with three phosphate groups, hence the name adenosine triphosphate. When energy is needed inside a cell, the end phosphate breaks away, creating a chemical reaction. Once all three phosphates have been released, the adenosine returns to the power generation unit so that it can be recharged with three more phosphates.

The term *machine* is most appropriate to describe the cell's power generation unit because it has moving parts. The generation unit that creates the ATPs has a crankshaft that spins around in a circular motion. During this process, oxygen allows the power plants to produce 36 ATPs from a single sugar molecule, and without oxygen, they can only create two ATPs from every sugar molecule. Because oxygen has such a powerful attraction to electrons, an abundance of oxygen allows your body to create more energy.

When a man walks, runs, bikes or jogs for 30 minutes a day, it strengthens his cardiovascular system and forces his lungs to produce and deliver more oxygen. When more oxygen is delivered to the power generation units, it allows his cells to create more energy. That's why people who work out on a regular basis have more energy. They can accomplish simple tasks around the house without ever growing tired. Their lungs have been trained to produce more oxygen, which in turn allows their cells to deliver more energy.

Exercise Releases Endorphins

Not only will regular exercise allow your cells to produce more energy, but it will also cause your body to release endorphins that burn fat and eliminate depression. A good example of how exercise can eliminate depression comes from a man named Scott. At one point in Scott's life, he was working at a great job and living in an expensive home, but after experiencing a financial downturn, his wife filed for divorce. After selling his home for less money than it was worth, Scott found himself depressed and living in his parent's basement.

Scott's depression continued spiraling downward until he hit bottom one day and started thinking about suicide. Because Scott didn't want to end his life or turn to drugs, alcohol or antidepressant medication to make himself feel better, he started going to the gym. The social environment at the gym provided a healthy atmosphere for Scott to meet new friends. It also allowed the subtle smiles and greetings that he received to change his attitude.

Within the first few months of working out, Scott began to notice major changes in his life. He was surprised by the profound affect that exercise could have on his mental, emotional and physical well-being. When Scott forced his body to perform cardiovascular exercise, his body decreased the amount of the harmful stress hormone cortisol that it had been producing and began releasing powerful mood-altering endorphins, including adrenaline, serotonin and dopamine.

Because endorphins are the body's natural painkillers, Scott began to enjoy the same kind of natural high that long-distance runners experience. When Scott's brain started releasing powerful mood-altering endorphins, it created feelings of euphoria that quickly eliminated his depression.

In addition to receiving a euphoric runner's high, Scott's body also started producing hormones that suppressed his appetite, increased his metabolism and told his liver to stop converting extra glucose into fatty acid. Within a very short amount of time, Scott was able to lose weight, increase his energy levels, sleep better at night and eliminate depression from his life.

Eliminating Back Problems

Another reason why physical exercise is important comes from a young woman named Marsha who had been experiencing back pain for many years. Because the pain was so bad that she could barely move at times, Marsha was considering an operation that would fuse the vertebra in her spine together. As she pondered the potential risks of the operation, she began to worry and started looking for better alternatives.

By studying the human anatomy, it's easy to see why Marsha had been experiencing so much pain. Her spine was comprised of tiny disks stacked one on top of the other. The only counterbalance to this design was her stomach muscles. By working out on a regular basis, Marsha could strengthen her stomach muscles and create a stronger support for her upper body weight.

To receive the healing that Marsha desired, she needed to strengthen her stomach muscles even though she was still experiencing a lot of back pain. The process took several months, but through persistence and hard work, she was able to strengthen her abdomen and lower back muscles to the point where they began to take pressure off her spine. As soon as the pressure was released, the swelling around her disks decreased, her nerves began to relax, and within a few months, she made a complete recovery.

In the event that you are experiencing lower back pain, the only effective way to deal with the situation would be to start working out on a regular basis. There are many abdominal and lower back exercises that you can do in the privacy of your own home. All you need to do is conduct an Internet search using the keywords, "exercises to strengthen lower back and abdomen muscles."

Increased Weight Loss

Another woman named Gloria wanted to work out at her local gym, but because of her current health condition, she eventually gave up on the possibility. Gloria had struggled with weight loss her entire life. The amazing part of Gloria's situation was her determination and persistence to eat only one meal per day.

Gloria began the day by drinking decaffeinated coffee and a lot of water. Even though she became hungry around 11 a.m., she fought the urge to eat until she got off work. When Gloria returned home, she would consume a large meal, and after watching several hours of television, she would go to bed for the evening.

Because Gloria's body didn't need thousands of calories right before she went to sleep, her liver would convert her entire dinner into fatty acids, which it made available for her to use the following morning. In the event that Gloria's body didn't consume all the fatty acids the next day, it would eventually be converted into saturated fat.

Another problem with eating a large meal right before going to bed was that Gloria's body had to spend at lot of time and energy digesting the food and converting it into fatty acids before it could perform the more important functions of removing toxins, fighting disease and rebalancing her internal chemistry.

In order to solve these health issues, Gloria needed to stop eating a large meal in the evening and start eating a healthy breakfast. The only problem was that Gloria was not hungry in the morning, and she was terrified of eating food during the day because it would only increase her cravings.

To begin the healing process, Gloria made a commitment to never eat past 2 p.m., with the exception of a small piece of fruit around dinnertime. When Gloria stopped eating at night, she found herself extremely hungry in the morning. Gloria was so hungry that she began eating four meals per day. Her first breakfast started early in the morning with a piece of fruit. Her second breakfast consisted of raw vegetables and grains, and her third breakfast consisted of vegetables with a good source of protein, such as eggs one morning and fat-free milk the next.

For lunch, Gloria would consume the same type of meal that she normally ate for dinner, except she started eating more raw vegetables and less animal protein. In the event that Gloria needed a little extra energy in the evenings, she would eat a small piece of fruit for dinner. Because Gloria stopped eating a large meal right before going to bed, her body stopped producing fatty acids and she was able to sleep better at night.

Another benefit that Gloria discovered was that when she gave her body the nutrients it needed, at exactly the right time when her body needed them, her constant cravings for food decreased by 85 percent. Gloria was able to eat twice as much food as before, and she soon began losing a serious amount of weight.

Gloria was so excited about her newfound relationship with a healthy organic diet that she signed up for a membership at her local gym. When Gloria began working out on a regular basis, she was able to consume even more calories per day and still continued losing weight.

Two-Hour Workout Session

In an effort to keep your body in prime condition, you may want to consider visiting your local gym twice a week for a two-hour workout session. Although a two-hour workout may seem like a long time, if you force your body past its point of resistance, within a few short months, it will grow accustomed to the routine and will no longer stage a protest. A two-hour workout session (combined with prayer) twice a week will also transform your life with a stress-reducing time of peaceful mental relaxation.

Workout options at the gym include using the StairMaster, elliptical trainer, stationary bike, rowing machine, treadmill, free weights and other machines. In the event that you don't like going to the gym, there are many outdoor activities, including jogging, power walking, cycling, downhill skiing, cross-country skiing, snowshoeing, swimming, water skiing, wakeboarding, surfing, rock climbing, rollerblading, kickboxing, skateboarding, ice skating, playing tennis, volleyball, lacrosse, basketball, hockey or soccer.

In the event you don't like outdoor activities, there's racquetball, step aerobics, spinning classes, Jazzercise and salsa dancing. It's also possible to work out in the privacy of your home using popular videos such as the *10 Minute Solution: High Intensity Interval Training* or *Tony Horton's 10-Minute Trainer.*

An additional benefit of joining a gym would be the availability of a steam room or sauna. Spending 15 minutes in the steam room after a two-hour workout session is a great way to reward yourself while relaxing your muscles and alleviating any joint pain. A steam room will also help reduce stress, raise your metabolism, boost your immune system, remove deadly toxins from your body, improve your complexion and alleviate symptoms of a cold.

Regular exercise will strengthen your muscles, release hormones that burn fat, increase your lung's ability to produce oxygen, give you more energy, release mood-altering endorphins, generate feelings of euphoria and allow you to fall asleep faster and experience a deeper and more peaceful night's rest.

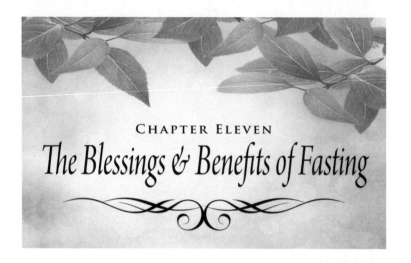

CHAPTER ELEVEN

The Blessings & Benefits of Fasting

One afternoon while God was walking through the garden, Eve rushed down the southern hillside to meet him. Crossing the cobblestone path near the stream, she fell to her knees as she approached the Lord, saying, "Please come quickly. Something's wrong with Sox. He usually comes to visit us before nightfall, but the past few days, we began to worry about him and went looking. We found him curled up in his den."

As God approached the rocky cliffs, Adam reached out to hold Eve's hand and said, "I have been trying to feed Sox, but he won't eat anything. Will you please help him?" As Adam was still speaking, the red fox peered out from between the rocks. After looking around, he slowly emerged, stretching forth his black paws and yawning as he proceeded.

Sox's reddish-white fur gradually faded into different shades of gray until it reached the tip of his black tail. His coat was normally thick and lush, but today it appeared straggly and matted. Sox eventually shook off the dust and fluffed up his fur as if wanting to make his best appearance before the King.

"He will be fine," God said. "I could perform a miracle healing, but it's best to allow his body to heal naturally."

"I think he ate some spoiled food," Eve said.

"I think you're right," God said. "But why are you trying to feed him when he's not hungry?"

"Well," Adam responded, as he looked down at Sox, "I guess, I wanted him to regain his strength so that everything would be okay."

"You know, Adam, it's best to allow animals their fast. I designed them that way. They instinctually know how to heal themselves. Sox doesn't want to eat because his body needs to conserve energy and resources to fight the infection."

"But I thought he might be hungry," Adam said.

"Sox can survive all week without eating anything, and so can you. Do you remember when you drank water from the duck pond? How you weren't hungry the following day?"

"Yes," Adam said.

"During that time, your body needed to rest and recover. It takes a lot of energy and internal resources to digest and assimilate nutrients from food. It's much easier for your body to use its stored energy reserves. That way, all of your body's internal resources can be focused on fighting the infection."

"I'm so happy Sox is going to be okay," Eve said.

"He will be fine," God said. "He only wants to go

back to sleep. Let's give him a few more days. Besides, it's getting late. If you walk back to the garden with me, I will share with you the benefits of fasting."

Burning Fat for Fuel

When the human body becomes infected with a virus, it needs all of its strength to fight the infection and doesn't want to waste valuable resources digesting food, especially when there's a vast storehouse of fat available that it can quickly convert to energy. This fat-burning process is called *ketosis* or *ketone production*. The human body usually burns glucose as its primary fuel source, but when a man stops eating for two days, his body will start burning fat as fuel.

When a man consumes a healthy diet of fresh fruits, vegetables, grains and seeds in the proper amounts when his body needs them, his digestive system can handle the workload, neutralizing toxins, removing waste and assimilating the valuable nutrients.

When a man consumes hydrogenated oils, processed foods and toxic chemicals, his digestive system can become overwhelmed. When there's not enough time to neutralize toxins and remove waste, his body will store the fat-soluble toxins inside of fat cells.

Not only do fat cells store toxins, but they also have a nucleus and the ability to release hormones. For example, one hormone called *leptin* controls the body's appetite and metabolism. Another hormone called *adiponectin* affects the body's sensitivity to insulin. When an excessive amount of fat cells produce too many hormones, it can wreak havoc on a person's internal chemistry.

One of the greatest benefits of fasting is that it allows the human body to naturally burn fat as fuel, and by doing so, eliminate the excessive hormones that fat cells produce. By removing excessive fat storage from your body, you will also be removing the fat-soluble toxins that are being stored inside those cells, and preventing those cells from mutating and becoming cancerous.

Internal House Cleaning

When a man starts fasting, the first few days will be the hardest. His blood sugar levels will drop, and he will usually feel irritable and cranky. After the first 24 hours have passed, his liver will tap into its emergency fuel reserve called *glycogen*. The liver stores enough glycogen for about 12 hours of energy, and after it has been consumed, the man's body will start burning fat for fuel. Once his body starts burning fat, his liver will replenish his emergency fuel reserves and he will start feeling better.

After 36 hours have passed, the man's digestive system will begin the process of shutting down. His liver will stop producing bile, and any extra bile will be stored in his gallbladder. The man's pancreas will stop producing digestive enzymes, and the cells in his stomach lining will stop producing hydrochloric acid. During this time, he man's digestive system will be able to rest, and when it restarts, his internal chemistry will be restored to its natural settings.

The third day of the fast is a great relief for many people, because that's when they experience a spiritual high. On the third day of the fast, the brain will release endorphins (the body's natural pain killers) that will make a person feel more empowered. The endorphins will also allow a person to think more clearly. During this time, many people experience what they describe as a *spiritual high.*

In an attempt to acquire protein during the fast, the human body will begin seeking out all nonessential cellular material such as tumors, degenerative tissues, waste products in the blood, buildup around the joints and any other nonessential cellular debris that can be broken down into amino acids. This internal house-cleaning process is why fasting produces such great health benefits.

Health Benefits of Fasting

A good example of the health benefits that fasting produces comes from a man named John who suffered from rheumatoid arthritis for many years. In John's case, there was an excessive amount of dead cellular debris in his joints that was causing painful inflammation. Because John didn't want to take painkillers that would damage his liver, he began looking for an alternative that would address the root cause of the problem. In his research, John came across a number of studies establishing fasting as an effective treatment for both osteoarthritis and rheumatoid arthritis.

Fasting has the power to heal arthritis (and many other medical conditions) because when the human body is starved for fuel, it will start cannibalizing all nonessential tissue. When looking for nonessential tissue, it will start consuming tumors and abnormal growths. Once all the tumors have been removed and used for fuel, the body will start cleaning out all dead cellular debris that has accumulated inside the arteries over the years (causing high blood pressure) and convert that material into the amino acids it needs to support more important functions.

In John's case, when his body was being starved for fuel, it started cleaning out all the dead cellular debris in his joints to use as fuel. John's healing process took over a year to complete, because he started out very slowly. At first, he just skipped lunch one afternoon to see what would happen. Next, he went all day without eating. After starting off slowly and fasting for several days on many different occasions, John's body was finally able to remove the excessive buildup in his joints and repair the damaged cartilage. Today, John is pain free and considers himself completely healed of rheumatoid arthritis.

In another medically supervised situation, over a hundred people with high blood pressure began fasting three days by eating only fruits and vegetables. Next, the participants transitioned to a 10-day water fast, followed by a post-fast where they ate a low-fat vegetarian diet for seven days. By the end of the program, 90 percent of the participants achieved blood pressure levels less than 140/90. Those who began the fast with blood pressure over 180/110 had an average reduction rate of 60/17. All the participants that were taking high blood pressure medication prior to the fast were able to discontinue using it after fasting.[1]

Other health benefits of fasting include the ability to experience a peaceful night's sleep, more energy, a newfound desire to change poor dietary habits, increased weight loss, an improved sense of vision and hearing, a reduction in allergies and headaches, clearer skin, the elimination of asthma, hay fever and fibromyalgia, lower cholesterol and less chronic joint pain.

Seven-Day Blender Fast

One easy way to start fasting only requires a blender with some fruit and vegetables. To begin the fast, all you need to do is set aside a specific amount of time. If you have never fasted before, you may want to start with just one day. Those with more experience and the acquired discipline can set aside a full week. For breakfast, all you need to do is pour a cup of water in the blender and drop in some fruit. Options for fruit smoothies would include an apple, two sticks of celery and a cucumber.

After enjoying a fruit smoothie for breakfast, repeat the process for lunch and dinner, but instead of using fruit, switch over to raw vegetables. For lunch, you may want to try a tomato, three stalks of kale and two carrots. For dinner, try a cucumber, green bell pepper and spinach. Just pour a little water in your blender and add the vegetables a few pieces at a time.

It's also possible to use one vegetable at a time, for example, kale and water, then a few hours later, try some carrots and water. A peeled grapefruit (or two oranges) with a little water in the blender is an excellent way to start the day. Just make sure you drink plenty of water during the fast and take some organic food-sourced vitamins.

Another option would be to add a little protein to your juice along with some omega-3 and omega-6 fatty acids. This is very easily accomplished by adding a few tablespoons of chia seeds or ground flax seeds to the blender. Three bananas and some raw walnuts make an excellent smoothie. You may also want to try carrots, beetroot and chia seeds.

Preparations for Fasting

The best way to prepare for a fast is by slowly decreasing the amount of food you eat a few days prior. The longer and more intense period that you plan to fast, the more time you will want to spend in preparation. If you are planning to fast a few days on strictly water, it may be helpful to spend the first few days eating raw fruits and vegetables, then transition over to a blender fast for two days, and then revert to mostly water with a little fruit juice.

When breaking a water-only fast, you will want to revert back to fruit and vegetable juice for at least a day and then slowly transition back to eating raw fruits and vegetables. When returning to a normal diet, you will want to be very careful by choosing foods that contain pure and simple ingredients. If you try breaking a week-long fast with a spicy-hot burrito or imitation applesauce that's loaded with high fructose corn syrup and preservatives, it will probably cause stomach cramps and indigestion.

If you're a regular coffee drinker, it would also be helpful to slowly wean yourself off caffeine a few days prior to fasting in an attempt to avoid headaches during the fast. In the event that you're fasting longer than a week, it will be helpful to maintain your regular exercise and workout routine, except at a slower and more relaxed pace.

Another consideration for longer fasts would involve your colon's health. Many health professionals recommend one or two enemas during a longer fast, especially if the patient is feeling constipated. An inexpensive method for enemas involves buying a hot water bottle at your local pharmacy that includes a plastic hose designed for that purpose. All you need to do is follow the instructions on the package.

Another consideration would be to get plenty of sleep during your fast. In the event that you experience flu-like symptoms during the fast, they are usually caused by all the fat-soluble toxins that are being purged from your body. When this occurs, many people will experience stronger-smelling urine, a thick white coat on their tongue, and unpleasant underarm odor. All these symptoms are good signs that your body is effectively removing cancer-causing toxins that were being stored inside of fat cells.

Not only is it important to drink a lot of water while fasting, but it's equally important to continue drinking a lot of water after you break the fast. Drinking a lot of water during the fast will help your body remove toxins, and although you might not feel thirsty after breaking the fast, your body could still be burning toxic fat and creating more uric acid or other waste products than normal.

Another advantage to the blender fast is that you don't have to remove all the food from your house or buy a lot of expensive pasteurized and commercially processed juice. All you need to do is stop cooking grains and leave the animal protein in the freezer. If your countertops have been stocked with fresh fruits and your refrigerator is loaded with vegetables, you should be able to transition back and forth between your regular diet and the blender fast very easily.

Greater Spiritual Discipline

Fasting is also a powerful tool to develop greater spiritual discipline. A good example on how this process works comes from a woman named Jane who used to get cranky when she was hungry. Although Jane loved her children dearly and would never want to hurt them, when her blood sugar levels dropped, she would become agitated and lash out at her kids.

Her breaking point came late one Saturday afternoon when she was driving home after spending the day in the mountains. Jane hadn't stopped to eat lunch, and after running a few errands, her kids started fighting. Because the slightest annoyance would set Jane off, she started yelling at her kids, saying things that she deeply regretted.

During this time, several women from Jane's Bible study group started to explore the benefits of fasting. After discussing the topic in their group, Jane decided to give it a try. As soon as she skipped her first meal, her body threw a fit and she was immediately confronted with a lack of spiritual discipline.

At this point, Jane had a choice to make: Would she put her fleshly desires aside and continue fasting? Or would her fleshly desires win the battle and influence her actions? Because Jane desired a deeper relationship with God and a greater amount of spiritual discipline, she continued to fast. On the third day of her fast, her digestive system shut down and her brain started releasing pain-killing endorphins. As soon as Jane reached the third day of the fast, she found herself on a spiritual high.

A good example of the battle between Jane's flesh and her spirit has been described in Galatians 5:16–17, which says, *Live by the Spirit, I say, and do not gratify the desires of the flesh. For what the flesh desires is opposed to the Spirit, and what the Spirit desires is opposed to the flesh; for these are opposed to each other, to prevent you from doing what you want.*

After fasting on several different occasions, Jane began to grow tremendously in her relationship with the Lord. She soon acquired the ability to remain Spirit-filled and exhibited the fruits of the Spirit even when she was hungry. After acquiring a greater amount of spiritual discipline, Jane is now a changed woman with a newfound desire to serve the Lord in ministry.

Biblical Examples of Fasting

When Moses ascended to the top of Mount Sinai to receive the Ten Commandments from God, he fasted 40 days and nights. According to Exodus 34:28, *He was there with the Lord forty days and forty nights; he neither ate bread nor drank water.*

In 1 Kings 19:5–8, an angel of the Lord touched the prophet Elijah, who was asleep under a tree, and said, *"Get up and eat." He looked, and there at his head was a cake baked on hot stones, and a jar of water. He ate and drank, and lay down again.*

The angel of the Lord came a second time, touched him, and said, "Get up and eat, otherwise the journey will be too much for you." He got up, and ate and drank; then he went in the strength of that food forty days and forty nights to Horeb the mount of God.

When King Nebuchadnezzar placed several young men from Israel in his service, *Daniel resolved that he would not defile himself with the royal rations of food and wine. The palace master said to Daniel, "I am afraid of my lord the king; he has appointed your food and your drink. If he should see you in poorer condition than the other young men of your own age, you would endanger my head with the king."²*

Daniel responded by saying, *"Please test your servants for ten days. Let us be given vegetables to eat and water to drink. You can then compare our appearance with the appearance of the young men who eat the royal rations, and deal with your servants according to what you observe." So he agreed to this proposal and tested them for ten days.³*

At the end of ten days it was observed that they appeared better and fatter than all the young men who had been eating the royal rations. So the guard continued to withdraw their royal rations and the wine they were to drink, and gave them vegetables.⁴

According to Luke 2:37, there was a widow named Anna who *never left the temple but worshiped there with fasting and prayer night and day.*

In Acts 13:2–3, when the disciples *were worshiping the Lord and fasting, the Holy Spirit said, "Set apart for me Barnabas and Saul for the work to which I have called them." Then after fasting and praying they laid their hands on them and sent them off.*

Spiritual Benefits of Fasting

Drawing closer to God is another powerful benefit of fasting. Although Adam and Eve could personally commune with God in the garden during the time of the evening breeze, today we need to spend more time and effort seeking the Lord.

We need to make God a top priority in our lives and spend quality time and serious effort pursuing our relationship with him. Seeking a deeper relationship with the Lord through prayer and fasting is extremely powerful, because God already wants to commune with his beloved children.

When we set aside an entire week to pursue God through prayer and fasting, the Lord will honor our request and interact with us in profoundly new and miraculous ways.

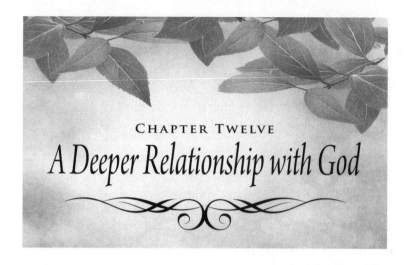

CHAPTER TWELVE
A Deeper Relationship with God

One day while God was walking through the garden during the time of the evening breeze, he approached a pond to inspect elements of his microscopic creation. Several thousand amoebas were maneuvering in the water in an attempt to capture prey.

Although these tiny creatures are commonly referred to as *single-celled* organisms, they are extremely complex. For example, amoebas have the ability to change their shape to surround and engulf prey. They also have a nucleus that contains DNA and chromosomes that control their growth and reproductive functions.

As God looked deep into the water, he noticed one very large amoeba that had been stalking a smaller paramecium for several hours. The unsuspecting paramecium didn't realize the danger until it was too late. The amoeba kept changing its shape, slowly and carefully. Once the paramecium was completely surrounded, the amoeba deployed acid through its food vacuole that broke the paramecium down into substance that could be absorbed into its cytoplasm for nourishment.

After digesting the paramecium for lunch, the amoeba excreted the excess water and waste through his contractile vacuole and spoke to the Lord, saying, "I want to evolve into something more important."

"You have been assigned an important role in my creation," God said. "It's your job to keep the pond clean, free from bacteria, algae and decaying plant matter."

"But I want your job!" the amoeba said. "I want to rule the universe."

"That's very interesting," God said. "Are you up for the challenge?"

"I'm ready," the amoeba said.

"If you can draft a genetic blueprint explaining exactly how you plan to evolve, I will consider transforming your life into something more advanced," God said.

"What do you mean by 'genetic blueprint'?" the amoeba asked.

"You have a very impressive porous membrane," God said. "Your outer shell allows you to absorb oxygen from the water. When the pond dries up, you have been given the ability to secrete a protective covering over your membrane until the conditions are more favorable. But if you plan to evolve into a human, you will need a different type of skin, arms, legs, lungs and optical vision."

"What's 'optical vision'?" the amoeba asked.

"Good point," God said. "How can a single-celled

organism that has no knowledge of vision create the extremely complex system of nerves and muscles that allows the eyes to focus and display visual images?"

"What do you mean by 'visual images'?" the amoeba asked.

"A good example comes from a video surveillance camera," God said. "When humans invent surveillance cameras, they will have the ability to auto-focus and rotate. The visual images will be displayed on video monitors. Because it would not be possible for mammals to have an external video monitor mounted on the side of their heads, the image would need to be automatically displayed in their consciousness."

"Wow," the amoeba said, "visual images that automatically appear."

"All you need to do is draft the genetic code that allows billions of cells to work together in perfect harmony. Some cells will need to form the cornea, iris, pupil and retina, while others would need to send electrical impulses to the brain to create perfectly focused images displayed automatically."

"I would really like to assume your role as ruler of the universe, but this challenge is way too difficult," the amoeba said. "Please give me something simpler."

"Maybe you could ask the tadpole for assistance," God said. "If you are planning to mutate into the frog's larva, maybe one of your tailed aquatic friends could offer some assistance."

"No way! I'm scared of those guys," the amoeba

said. "They have been known to eat hundreds of amoeba for lunch."

"If you are planning to morph into an tadpole that will develop into a frog, and if the frog plans to morph into a monkey, then maybe you could ask the baboon for help."

"Pretty please," the amoeba said.

"Okay, here's a simpler design issue to solve," God said. "The human heart and lungs need to deliver a constant supply of oxygen to trillions of hungry cells, even when that person is unconscious or sleeping. If you can draft the genetic language to accomplish this function, you can assume my role as Creator of the universe."

"That's way too difficult," the amoeba said. "I still want to be God. Please ask me a simpler question on a smaller scale, something concerning just one cell."

"Very well," God said. "As you know, single-celled organisms reproduce by copying their nucleus and splitting themselves in half. Because the human reproductive system is more complex, you would need to morph in such a way as to create both male and female species. If you didn't split yourself in half in just the right way, your offspring wouldn't be able to reproduce at all."

"I will work out those details later," the amoeba said. "Just ask the question!"

"In the male reproductive system, a sperm cell has a tail made of eukaryotic cilium that allows it to swim a tenth of an inch per minute. How does that cell accomplish this?"

"You're right," the amoeba said. "I will return to my assigned role in life to accomplish your purpose and plan. You have created me to digest algae, bacteria and dead plant matter. I will do my best to keep your pond in pristine condition."

Acknowledging God's Existence

The first step in developing a deeper relationship with the Lord would be to acknowledge his existence. Once God makes himself known to a man, his spiritual eyes will be opened, and from that point forward, he can start developing an authentic relationship with the Almighty.

In the event that you have never had an encounter with God, all you need to do is seek the Lord with all your heart and he will make himself very real to you. According to Proverbs 8:17, the Lord says, *"I love those who love me, and those who seek me diligently find me."* When you seek the Lord with all your heart, he will manifest his power and presence in your life.

To begin this process, you may want to start with a simple prayer as follows: *Dear Heavenly Father, although I have never had an encounter with you, I want to know you more intimately so that I may accomplish your will in my life. Please make yourself very real to me, so that after I experience your divine presence, I may do my best to love and serve you, both now and forever more.*

Protection from Evil

One reason why many people fail to acknowledge God's existence is that they are unwilling to surrender the lordship of their lives to anything other than themselves. Once a man acknowledges God's existence, it automatically obligates him to seek after his Creator. Because many individuals want to be their own god and follow their own ways, they are unwilling to enter into an authentic relationship with a perfectly holy God who may require a few lifestyle changes, including the acknowledgment of sin and a need to comply with his laws.

Although a perfectly holy God will require his beloved children to acknowledge, confess and repent of their sins, the process of sanctification offers many important benefits, including the protection from evil. Our need for protection from evil was first disclosed in the Garden of Eden when the serpent tempted Adam and Eve. The problem started before the world began when one of the highest-ranking angels started a rebellion.

According to Revelation 12:7–9, *war broke out in heaven; Michael and his angels fought against the dragon. The dragon and his angels fought back, but they were defeated, and there was no longer any place for them in heaven. The great dragon was thrown down, that ancient serpent, who is called the Devil and Satan, the deceiver of the whole world—he was thrown down to the earth, and his angels were thrown down with him.*

After Satan and a vast army of fallen angels were cast out of heaven, they started a deadly assault against humanity. Knowing that a perfectly holy God would not be able to tolerate sin and rebellion, they devised a plan. The first temptation occurred when the serpent seduced Adam and Eve with a piece of fruit. In Matthew 4:1–3, we see Satan tempting Jesus with a loaf of bread. In Luke 22:31, Satan demanded to sift Peter like wheat.

According to John 10:10, the devil has only one purpose, *to steal and kill and destroy.*

We also learn from Scripture that Satan, along with his vast army of fallen angels, have the ability to cause demonic illness. In Job 2:7, Satan *inflicted loathsome sores on Job from the sole of his foot to the crown of his head.* In Matthew 17:14–18, there was a boy who suffered from epilepsy, a chronic nervous disorder affecting muscular control and consciousness. After Jesus cast out the demon, the boy made a complete recovery.

In Luke 13:11–13, there was *a woman with a spirit that had crippled her for eighteen years. She was bent over and was quite unable to stand up straight. When Jesus saw her, he called her over and said, "Woman, you are set free from your ailment." When he laid his hands on her, immediately she stood up straight and began praising God.*

After Jesus healed the woman, the leaders of the synagogue became indignant because she had been cured on the Sabbath. After Jesus addressed their concerns, he disclosed the source of the woman's infirmity in Luke 13:16, by saying, *"And ought not this woman, a daughter of Abraham whom Satan bound for eighteen long years, be set free from this bondage on the Sabbath day?"*

In the event that you have been suffering from some strange and mysterious illness that no doctor can accurately diagnose or treat, there's great hope and healing available through Jesus. One of the most important reasons for becoming a Christian is that it changes your eternal status. You will be able to transition away from the kingdom of darkness and into the marvelous light.

When you become an authentic Christian, the Holy

Spirit will reside deep within your heart. God's Spirit will begin the process of transforming your life. You will become a child of the King, a new creation in Christ. You will have a newfound strength to resist the devil's temptations. Once your obedience in Christ is complete, you will be able to speak a simple command and the devil will flee from your presence.

Your Sins will be Forgiven

Another important reason for becoming a Christian is that your sins will be forgiven. According to Romans 6:23, *the wages of sin is death.* In the Old Covenant, when a man sinned he was allowed to place the penalty upon an innocent lamb. The lamb was slaughtered in the temple, and the lamb's blood atoned for the man's sin.

In the New Covenant, Jesus became the Lamb of God. Although Jesus lived a sinless life, he was condemned to die a violent death on the cross to make atonement for our sins. He was crucified, died and rose from the dead three days later. Now that Jesus has become the sacrificial Lamb of God, everybody has a choice to make: You can pay the death penalty yourself, or you can allow Jesus to pay the penalty on your behalf.

To explore this meaning further, it may be helpful to imagine what it would be like to stand in front of God's throne on the Day of Judgment. Picture what it would look like if all your sins were piled high upon your head—all the people you hurt and all your disobedient acts. Because God is perfectly holy, no form of sin, darkness or deception can ever enter his eternal presence. Although God is loving and doesn't want to see any of his children suffer, he is also a God of justice. When we sin, our actions harm other people. Because God loves the people whom our sins have harmed, he cannot simply turn his back on them and pretend they don't exist.

As you picture yourself standing in the heavenly courtroom awaiting judgment, ponder for a moment God's dilemma. Your sins, no matter how small, have harmed other people. All sin is an agreement with evil. Because you have sinned and fallen short of God's perfect standard of perfection, God needs to render a just verdict.

The very same people you have harmed may also be standing in the courtroom during your judgment. God cannot simply say, "Even though you hurt all these people, I'm going to ignore their pain and suffering." Such a statement may affirm God's love for you, but it would be in direct conflict with his perfectly holy and just nature.

It is for this reason that the penalty for sin is death. All have sinned and fallen short of God's standard of perfection, and now someone needs to pay the price. After God examines the evidence, he issues a guilty verdict, and requires the penalty to be paid in full.

Picture what it would be like to be escorted to a holding cell to await execution. Picture what it would be like to pay the death penalty for your sinful actions. The bars inside the jail cell are made of solid steel, the concrete walls are cold and dark, and there's no window or hope of escape.

Now picture Jesus the Messiah entering your cell dressed in sparkling white clothes. As you look into his eyes, it's apparent that he loves you very much. He reaches out his hand to take hold of your hand. He sits down next to you. Speaking in a soft voice, he draws near and says, "I will pay the penalty on your behalf. You can now go free."

Do you want to accept the Lord's offer? Will you allow Jesus to pay the death penalty on your behalf?

To accept the Lord's sacrifice, all you need to do is say a simple prayer from the sincerity of a contrite heart: *Dear Lord Jesus, I come before you sinful. My actions have harmed other people, and I'm truly sorry. Please forgive me. I realize that the penalty for sin is death, and I don't want to pay the penalty myself. I accept your sacrifice on the cross for the forgiveness of my sins. I place all my sinful actions upon your cross and ask to be washed clean. Please transform my life through the power of your Holy Spirit. I surrender my life into your service. Please help me to become the child of God that you have intended me to be.*

After you have accepted the Lord's sacrifice on the cross for the forgiveness of your sins, you now have direct access to God's throne. You can enter the heavenly courts anytime you want and speak directly to your Heavenly Father through prayer. According to Romans 8:26–27, the Holy Spirit will intercede on your behalf. You will be able to ask God questions about your life, and after sitting in silence and meditating on his will, you will be able to discern the answers. God will speak directly to your heart through the power of the Holy Spirit.

Living in Paradise with God

The ultimate reason to become a Christian would be to spend all eternity with God in paradise. Instead of recreating the same lush, tropical conditions that existed in the Garden of Eden, God has an even better plan. According to the book of Revelation, God is planning to build an incredible city that will emit *the glory of God and a radiance like a very rare jewel, like jasper, clear as crystal.*[1]

According to Revelation 21:21, the streets surrounding the city will be paved *with pure gold, transparent as glass.* The city will not have any temples, churches or synagogues because the city's center of worship will be *the Lord God the Almighty and the Lamb. And the city has no need of sun or moon to shine on it, for the glory of God is its light, and its lamp is the Lamb. The nations will walk by its light, and the kings of the earth will bring their glory into it. Its gates will never be shut by day—and there will be no night there.*[2]

The heavenly city will also have a river of life *bright as crystal, flowing from the throne of God and of the Lamb through the middle of the street of the city. On either side of the river is the tree of life with its twelve kinds of fruit, producing its fruit each month; and the leaves of the tree are for the healing of the nations.*[3] *But nothing unclean will enter it, nor anyone who practices abomination or falsehood, but only those who are written in the Lamb's book of life.*[4]

You will also have the opportunity to live in harmony with Adam and Eve and all the other Godly men and women from centuries past. According to the Book of

Revelation, the dead will be raised to life, and everybody will stand before God's throne to give an account for their actions. In the event that your name is written in the Book of Life, you will be able to enter the heavenly city along with the rest of God's beloved children.

There will not be any more pain, sickness or disease. God will *wipe every tear from their eyes. Death will be no more; mourning and crying and pain will be no more.*[5]

You will be able to live with God in paradise for all eternity.

Notes

Chapter One
Living in Paradise with God

1. Genesis 1:7.
2. The Geological Society of America, "Raising Giant Insects to Unravel Ancient Oxygen," (October 29, 2010): http://www.geosociety.org/news/pr/10-60.htm.
3. Genesis 3:1.
4. Genesis 3:2–3.
5. Genesis 3:4–5.
6. Genesis 3:6.
7. Ibid.
8. Genesis 3:8–9.
9. Genesis 3:10.
10. Genesis 3:11.
11. Genesis 3:12.
12. Genesis 3:13.
13. Ibid.
14. Genesis 3:22–23.
15. Genesis 3:21.

16. Genesis 6:5–6.

17. Genesis 6:13–14.

18. Genesis 6:17–18.

19. Genesis 7:11.

20. Genesis 6:17 & 19.

21. Genesis 9:1 & 3–4.

22. National Cancer Institute—United States Department of Health and Human Services, "Cancer Statistics," (Accessed January 10, 2016): http://www.cancer.gov/about-cancer/what-is-cancer/statistics.

23. World Health Organization, "Cancer," (February 2015): http://www.who.int/mediacentre/factsheets/fs297/en.

Chapter Two
First Consideration—Limit Salt

1. World Health Organization, "Cardiovascular Diseases," (January 2015): http://www.who.int/mediacentre/factsheets/fs317/en.

2. *The New England Journal of Medicine,* "Global Sodium Consumption and Death from Cardiovascular Causes," (August 14, 2014): http://www.nejm.org/doi/full/10.1056/NEJMoa1304127.

3. American Heart Association, "Shaking the Salt Habit," (May 18, 2015): http://www.heart.org/HEARTORG/Conditions/HighBloodPressure/PreventionTreatmentofHighBloodPressure/Shaking-the-Salt-Habit_UCM_303241_Article.jsp#.VowQk1KpGHM.

4. National Institutes of Health—Office of Dietary Supplements, "Fact Sheet for Consumers," (Accessed January 10, 2016): https://ods.od.nih.gov/factsheets/Iodine-Consumer.

Chapter Three
Second Consideration—Avoid Fat

1. United States Food and Nutrition Board—Institute of Medicine, "Dietary Reference Intakes for Energy, Carbohydrate, Fiber, Fat, Fatty Acids, Cholesterol, Protein, and Amino Acids," (Accessed January 10, 2016): http://www.nap.edu/read/10490/chapter/1.

2. American Nutrition Association, "Why is American Milk Banned in Europe," (Accessed January 10, 2016): http://americannutritionassociation.org/toolsandresources/milk-america%25C3%25A2%25E2%2582%25AC%25E2%2584%25A2s-health-problem.

3. United States Food and Drug Administration, "Final Determination Regarding Partially Hydrogenated Oils—Removing Trans Fat," (June 16, 2015): http://www.fda.gov/Food/IngredientsPackagingLabeling/FoodAdditivesIngredients/ucm449162.htm.

4. Center for Science in the Public Interest, "The Problems With Olestra," (Accessed January 10, 2016): https://www.cspinet.org/olestra/11cons.html.

Chapter Four
Third Consideration—No Sweets

1. Ben & Jerry's Homemade Inc., "New York Super Fudge Chunk," (Accessed January 10, 2016): http://www.benjerry.com/flavors/new-york-super-fudge-chunk-ice-cream. Ben & Jerry's is a registered trademark of Unilever.

2. Doctor Joseph Mercola, "Aspartame: By Far the Most Dangerous Substance Added to Most Foods Today," (November 6, 2011): http://articles.mercola.com/sites/articles/archive/2011/11/06/aspartame-most-dangerous-substance-added-to-food.aspx.

Chapter Five
Toxic Chemicals & Preservatives

1. United States National Library of Medicine—National Institutes of Health, "Sulfites—a food and drug administration review of recalls and reported adverse events," (August 2004): http://www.ncbi.nlm.nih.gov/pubmed/15330554.

2. United States Environmental Protection Agency, "Nitrates and Nitrites," (May 22, 2007): http://archive.epa.gov/region5/teach/web/pdf/nitrates_summary.pdf.

3. World Health Organization—International Agency for Research on Cancer, "Carrageenan," (Volume 31, 1983): http://www.inchem.org/documents/iarc/vol31/carrageenan.html.

4. "Coca-Cola" is a registered trademark of The Coca-Cola Company.

5. Live Science, "Does Coca-Cola Contain Cocaine," (December 16, 2013): http://www.livescience.com/41975-does-coca-cola-contain-cocaine.html.

6. The Coca-Cola Company, "The Secret Is Out: Coca-Cola's Formula Is at the World of Coca-Cola," (October 16, 2012): http://www.coca-colacompany.com/stories/the-secret-is-out-coca-colas-formula-is-at-the-world-of-coca-cola.

7. Center for Science in the Public Interest, "FDA Urged to Prohibit Carcinogenic 'Caramel Coloring,'" (February 16, 2011): http://www.cspinet.org/new/201102161.html.

8. United States Food and Drug Administration, "What is the meaning of 'natural' on the label of food," (Accessed January 10, 2016): http://www.fda.gov/aboutfda/transparency/basics/ucm214868.htm.

9. Natural News Network, "True fact: A common ingredient in commercial breads is derived from human hair harvested in China," (June 16, 2011): http://www.naturalnews.com/032718_L-cysteine_commercial_bread.html.

Chapter Six
A Healthy Diet of Organic Plants

1. Monsanto Company, "Glyphosate and Roundup Brand Herbicides," (Accessed January 10, 2016): http://www.monsanto.com/glyphosate/pages/default.aspx.

2. National Center for Biotechnology Information, "Soybean genetic transformation: A valuable tool for the functional study of genes and the production of agronomically improved plants," (December 18, 2012): http://www.ncbi.nlm.nih.gov/pmc/articles/PMC3571417/.

3. International Service for the Acquisition of Agri-biotech Applications, "GM Approval Database," (Accessed January 10, 2016): http://www.isaaa.org/gmapprovaldatabase.

4. United States Food and Drug Administration, "AquAdvantage Salmon," (Accessed January 10, 2016): http://www.fda.gov/AnimalVeterinary/DevelopmentApprovalProcess/GeneticEngineering/GeneticallyEngineeredAnimals/ucm280853.htm.

Chapter Seven
Evaluating Your Environment

1. FracFocus Chemical Disclosure Registry, "What Chemicals are Used," (Accessed January 10, 2016): http://fracfocus.org/chemical-use/what-chemicals-are-used.

2. Environmental Working Group, "National Drinking Water Database," (Accessed January 10, 2016): http://www.ewg.org/tap-water.

3. Centers for Disease Control and Prevention, "Community Water Fluoridation," (Accessed January 10, 2016): http://www.cdc.gov/fluoridation/basics/index.htm.

4. *American Journal of Public Health,* "The Role of Skin Absorption as a Route of Exposure for Volatile Organic Compounds (VOCs) in Drinking Water," (May 1984): http://ajph.aphapublications.org/doi/pdf/10.2105/AJPH.74.5.479.

5. *Journal of Inorganic Biochemistry,* "Are Aluminum-Containing Antiperspirants Contributing To Breast Cancer In Women?" (October 17, 2011): http://articles.mercola.com/sites/articles/archive/2011/10/17/aluminum-containing-antiperspirants-contribute-breast-cancer.aspx.

6. United States Environmental Protection Agency, "Cleaning Up a Broken CFL," (Accessed January 10, 2016): http://www.epa.gov/cfl/cleaning-broken-cfl#instructions.

7. Canadian Cancer Society, "Phthalates," (Accessed January 10, 2016): http://www.cancer.ca/en/prevention-and-screening/be-aware/harmful-substances-and-environmental-risks/phthalates/?region=on.

8. World Health Organization—International Agency for Research on

Cancer, "Styrene," (Volume 82, 2002): http://www.inchem.org/documents/iarc/vol82/82-07.html.

9. *International Journal of Electrochemical Science,* "Risk Assessment of Using Aluminum Foil in Food Preparation," (May 1, 2012): http://www.electrochemsci.org/papers/vol7/7054498.pdf.

10. World Health Organization—International Agency for Research on Cancer, "Carcinogenicity of combined hormonal contraceptives and combined menopausal treatment," (September 2005): http://www.who.int/reproductivehealth/publications/ageing/cocs_hrt_statement.pdf?ua=1.

Chapter Eight
The Lord's Dietary Restrictions

1. Genesis 4:6–7.

2. Genesis 4:8.

3. Ibid.

4. Genesis 4:9.

5. Ibid.

6. Genesis 4:10–12.

7. Genesis 4:16.

8. Genesis 9:5.

9. Leviticus 17:11 & 3:17.

10. United States Department of Defense, "Operation United Assistance at a Glance," (Accessed January 10, 2016): http://archive.defense.gov/home/features/2014/1014_ebola.

11. United States Department of Agriculture, "Swine Disease Information," (Accessed January 10, 2016): https://www.aphis.usda.gov/wps/portal/aphis/ourfocus/animalhealth/sa_animal_disease_information.

12. Leviticus 11:8.

13. Mark 7:5.

14. Mark 7:21–23.

15. Mark 7:14–15.

16. Mark 7:17–19.

17. United States Food and Drug Administration, "What You Need to Know About Mercury in Fish and Shellfish," (March 2004): http://www.fda.gov/Food/ResourcesForYou/Consumers/ucm110591.htm.

18. Environmental Working Group, "PCBs in Farmed Salmon—Test results show high levels of contamination," (July 31, 2003): http://www.ewg.org/research/pcbs-farmed-salmon.

19. University at Albany—State University of New York, "First Global Study Reveals Health Risks of Widely Eaten Farm Raised Salmon," (January 9, 2004): http://albany.edu/ihe/salmonstudy.

20. Bloomberg Business News, "Asian Seafood Raised on Pig Feces Approved for U.S. Consumers," (October 10, 2012): http://www.bloomberg.com/news/articles/2012-10-11/asian-seafood-raised-on-pig-feces-approved-for-u-s-consumers.
21. Ibid.

Chapter Nine
Honoring the Sabbath Day's Rest
1. Philippians 4:4–6 & 8.
2. Exodus 20:8–11.

Chapter Ten
The Importance of Physical Exercise
1. Genesis 2:7.

Chapter Eleven
The Blessings & Benefits of Fasting
1. Pomorski Medical University, "Medically Supervised Water-Only Fasting in the Treatment of Hypertension," (Accessed January 10, 2016): http://sci.pam.szczecin.pl/~fasting/download/fasting/articles/cardiovascular/hyperten.htm.
2. Daniel 1:8 & 10.
3. Daniel 1:12–14.
4. Daniel 1:15–16.

Chapter Twelve
A Deeper Relationship with God
1. Revelation 21:11.
2. Revelation 21:22–25.
3. Revelation 22:1–2.
4. Revelation 21:27.
5. Revelation 21:4.

Healing Power for the Heart
by Robert Abel

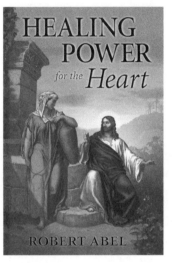

Do you feel distant from God's love? Are you searching for ultimate fulfillment in life?

Jesus came so that you may have life and have it more abundantly! He wants to heal all your wounds and fill your heart with his incredible love.

In this book, Robert Abel will show you how to establish a deeper and more passionate relationship with Jesus. The spiritual exercises on these life-giving pages have the power to break all forms of bondage in your life, and bring the Lord's healing power into all your traumatic past experiences.

Jesus wants to take you on an exciting adventure deep within the recesses of your soul. Embark upon the adventure of a lifetime. Open your heart and experience the fullness of God's extravagant love.

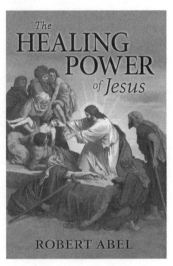

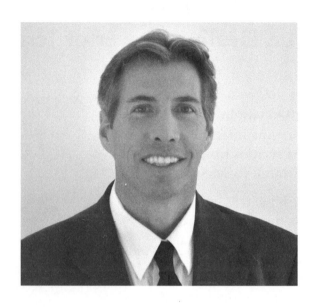

About the Author

Robert Abel's purpose and passion in life is speaking God's truth unto today's generation. He lives in Denver, Colorado, where he helps others heal through counseling sessions and healing seminars.

If you would like Robert to speak at your church, or if you would like to share your healing testimony, please contact **www.HealingPowerMinistries.com**

If you would like to participate in our ministry, please consider distributing copies of *Living in the Garden of Eden* to your friends and family. To purchase additional copies, please use the following information:

Number of Copies	Ministry Price
3	$25
6	$45
9	$55

These prices include tax and free shipping within the United States. For shipments to other countries, please contact us. Thank you for your generous support.

Mail your payment to:

Valentine Publishing House
Living in the Garden of Eden
P.O. Box 27422
Denver, Colorado 80227